V

# The Anxiety Cure for Kids

| DATE | | |
|---|---|---|
| | | |
| | | |
| | | |
| | | |
| | | |
| | | |
| | | |
| | | |
| | | |
| | | |
| | | |

6/09-8

Also by the authors

*The Anxiety Cure*

# The Anxiety Cure for Kids

## A Guide for Parents

Elizabeth DuPont Spencer, M.S.W.
Robert L. DuPont, M.D.
Caroline M. DuPont, M.D.

WILEY

John Wiley & Sons, Inc.

Published by John Wiley & Sons, Inc., Hoboken, New Jersey
Published simultaneously in Canada

Design and production by Navta Associates, Inc.

No part of this publication may be reproduced, stored in a retrieval system, or transmitted in any form or by any means, electronic, mechanical, photocopying, recording, scanning, or otherwise, except as permitted under Section 107 or 108 of the 1976 United States Copyright Act, without either the prior written permission of the Publisher, or authorization through payment of the appropriate per-copy fee to the Copyright Clearance Center, 222 Rosewood Drive, Danvers, MA 01923, (978) 750-8400, fax (978) 750-4470, or on the web at www.copyright.com. Requests to the Publisher for permission should be addressed to the Permissions Department, John Wiley & Sons, Inc., 111 River Street, Hoboken, NJ 07030, (201) 748-6011, fax (201) 748-6008, email: permcoordinator@wiley.com.

Limit of Liability/Disclaimer of Warranty: While the publisher and the author have used their best efforts in preparing this book, they make no representations or warranties with respect to the accuracy or completeness of the contents of this book and specifically disclaim any implied warranties of merchantability or fitness for a particular purpose. No warranty may be created or extended by sales representatives or written sales materials. The advice and strategies contained herein may not be suitable for your situation. You should consult with a professional where appropriate. Neither the publisher nor the author shall be liable for any loss of profit or any other commercial damages, including but not limited to special, incidental, consequential, or other damages.

For general information about our other products and services, please contact our Customer Care Department within the United States at (800) 762-2974, outside the United States at (317) 572-3993 or fax (317) 572-4002.

Wiley also publishes its books in a variety of electronic formats. Some content that appears in print may not be available in electronic books. For more information about Wiley products, visit our web site at www.wiley.com.

*Library of Congress Cataloging-in-Publication Data:*

Spencer, Elizabeth DuPont, date.
   The anxiety cure for kids : a guide for parents / Elizabeth DuPont
Spencer, Robert L. DuPont, Caroline M. DuPont.
      p. cm.
   Includes bibliographical references and index.
   ISBN 0-471-26361-3 (pbk.)
   1. Anxiety in children—Popular works. I. DuPont, Robert L., 1936-
II. DuPont, Caroline M., 1968- III. Title.
   RJ506.A58S66 2003
   618.92'85223—dc21

                                                      2002155888
Printed in the United States of America

10  9  8  7  6  5  4

This book is dedicated to anxious children and their parents.

Your suffering is our calling. We are inspired by the dream that overcoming anxiety problems during childhood will end the pain and disability of anxiety so that when anxious children become adults and care for their own children, this problem will be a distant but encouraging memory.

# CONTENTS

## PART THREE
## Beyond Anxiety

# FOREWORD

More children suffer from anxiety disorders than any other emotional disorder. Anxiety paralyzes a child's normal development and robs a child of the opportunities to experience the joys of youth. Children with anxiety disorders often have social, school, and family problems.

There has been recent recognition that childhood anxiety disorders are chronic and tend to persist into adulthood. Therefore, early identification and treatment of childhood anxiety disorders is critical. Attention has been focused on specific psychotherapies and medication as treatment options.

*The Anxiety Cure for Kids: A Guide for Parents* provides the missing essential ingredient to current treatment for anxious children. Parents are actively enlisted to assist with their child's treatment.

This book is written for parents and explains anxiety in children and its treatment in a meaningful and straightforward way. Using a Dragon to characterize anxiety and a Wizard to manage anxiety is elegantly simple and gives parents a useful means to understand and help their anxious child.

The most recent treatment research related to therapy and medication for children with anxiety disorders is presented in this book and is a basis for many of the clinical illustrations. Parents are given practical, step-by-step suggestions to help their child deal with and overcome anxiety.

The field is indebted to this family of mental health professionals who, in writing this book, have drawn upon their extensive knowledge and clinical expertise to provide a sage guide to parents whose children suffer from anxiety.

Karen Dineen Wagner, M.D., Ph.D.
Clarence Ross Miller Professor and Vice Chair
Department of Psychiatry and Behavioral Sciences
Director, Division of Child and Adolescent Psychiatry
University of Texas Medical Branch

# ACKNOWLEDGMENTS

This book exists because many people have helped us along the way. Our editor at Wiley, Thomas Miller, believed in us from the time he saw a draft of our first anxiety book. He urged us to extend our work by writing for parents and children. Thank you, Tom, for your support and guidance. Thank you also to our copy editor, Patricia Waldygo, and our production editor, Hope Breeman, for checking all the details.

Our families have challenged us to keep working to overcome anxiety problems using the ideas that we have found so successful in our personal and professional lives. Thank you for your love, Helen, Bill, Paul, Spence, Robert, David, and Colleen.

Many anxious patients and their families have educated and inspired us. We treasure our relationships with you. We are honored that you have chosen to let us into these personal, painful parts of your lives to offer our help.

Most especially we thank our colleagues who study and treat anxiety disorders. Without the thousands of researchers working to understand the biology and treatment of anxiety, a cure for anxiety would be impossible. Without the thousands more physicians and therapists who work every day with anxious people and their families, the treatment for anxiety would be useless. Thank you all for your ongoing work to help to solve this painful, puzzling, and fascinating human problem.

# A LETTER TO KIDS WITH ANXIETY PROBLEMS

Dear Young Reader:

This book is about being scared of being scared. You probably noticed that some kids are scared more than other kids are. Sometimes kids are scared even when most kids see nothing to be afraid of. Some people like to be scared, for example, when they ride a roller coaster at an amusement park or listen to a ghost story on Halloween. Of course, everyone is scared of something sometime. This is good! Being scared helps us when we are really in danger. Our bodies react quickly when we're afraid so that we can run fast to get away from things that scare us. Fear helps us get to someone who can help us.

But what about a kid who is scared of dogs and won't go to his friend's house because the friend has a dog? Or a kid who is too scared to even walk outside, because there *might* be a dog around? Or someone who stays up for hours past her bedtime because she is scared something bad will happen to her parents during the night? Kids are afraid of what might happen to them and to their parents. When kids are scared, they want their parents to help them feel safe. Being scared can feel extra scary when other people don't understand why you're scared! Sometimes it's hard to explain why you do things to keep yourself from being scared. Sometimes kids stay away from things that scare them or have to do things certain odd ways to make themselves feel safe. Being scared of being scared is called "anxiety." Having anxiety means that you worry about things that most kids don't worry about.

We think of anxiety as being like an imaginary Dragon in your head. The Dragon seems to be really scary. It can make you feel terribly afraid even when other kids are not upset. You should know that it's OK to feel scared.

This doesn't make you a bad person. Feeling scared doesn't have to limit what you do with your life. You can do everything you want to do, even if you feel scared. The Dragon can't really harm you. It can't make you sick. It wants you to think it can, but it doesn't have  that power. You can learn to tame the Dragon with help from the Wizard you also have in your own head. The Wizard will teach you powerful magic to tame the anxiety Dragon.

We, the authors, are two psychiatrists and a therapist, a father and two grown daughters with children of our own. We work together to help kids who have anxiety problems. This book has lots of stories about kids with anxiety. The kids' names have been changed to protect their privacy. Some stories are about kids we have seen recently, and some are about kids we saw so long ago, they're grown up now. All of these kids got better from the anxiety problems that brought them to us. By helping these kids, we learned everything that we'll teach you in this book. We're glad that we had the opportunity to learn from these kids: they were our teachers. We want you to learn from their stories, too.

You will need a Journal to write in, to describe how you get better from anxiety. This Journal will be your own how-to book about taming your Dragon. Your Journal is an important part of your Wizard magic. You  may want help in keeping your Journal. No matter how old you are, you may want to draw pictures to go along with the charts or stories you put in your Journal. Be creative. This is your own personal Journal. Make it your own by what you write and draw in it. We will give you many ideas about things other kids have done with their Journals.

Your Journal will help you now as you shrink your anxiety Dragon, and it will help you in the future if the Dragon comes back. Journals are especially useful because they are portable! If you are afraid of a roller coaster, you can take your Journal with you while you wait in line. Even when you go places alone, without the adult who knows how you are taming your Dragon, your Journal can be with you. Using the Wizard's magic in your Journal is the best way to remember how far you have come. Your own writing will show you how strong you have made your mind. The Wizard in your mind knows that the Dragon can't really hurt you.

You might be surprised to find out that there are many good things about having anxiety! Maybe you never thought of this before, because it feels bad to be scared when you don't understand why you're scared. We know that kids who are easily scared are really good kids. They can learn how to make their fears work for them instead of against them. The lessons in this book about being scared have helped a lot of other kids. We bet that they will help you, too.

Our book is addressed to your parents, who can become your best allies in helping tame the Dragon. Getting well is a challenge for your whole family. Use your family team to help you get free from the Dragon's prison. Good luck.

# Introduction and Guide to This Book

Welcome to an amazing world and to the upbeat story of a Dragon that is tamed by a Wizard. The Dragon uses the power of anxiety—fear and worry, upset stomachs, headaches, and intense self-doubt—to coax children into its prison. The Dragon can limit children's freedom to explore the world of opportunities all around them. This world is scary not only for children but for parents, too. The Dragon uses fear to control children.

The other imaginary character in this book is the Wizard, who teaches children and their parents magic to use every day to tame the Dragon. With this magic, which can be mastered with practice, parents and children can not only neutralize the Dragon's power but can also turn his attacks into positive opportunities for the whole family.

Part of each chapter, the Research Notes of Anxiety, provides you with useful facts about the modern understanding of anxiety, to put what you will learn into a scientific context. The two characters, the Wizard and the Dragon, will help you communicate your understanding to your anxious child. They will make this book easier to use. The Wizard and the Dragon, along with the Research Notes, are especially valuable because the ideas in this book are not obvious. The solutions to the anxiety puzzle are not easy to translate into the everyday life of your family. You will learn that your child's natural tendencies to flee from anxiety, to do the Dragon's bidding, are certain to lead your child even deeper into the Dragon's prison.

This book is written primarily for parents who are helping their children overcome anxiety problems. Our use of the Wizard and the Dragon could easily be misunderstood. These two characters are neither cartoons nor cute gimmicks for children. They help adults and children understand the devilishly cunning and baffling way that anxiety works. They also help parents and children talk about anxiety and learn how to overcome the negative impact of anxiety on their lives. Using the two characters creates a meaningful vocabulary and a format to discuss anxiety and its cure with children.

You will learn that your natural tendencies to criticize or to blame your child for anxiety-caused behaviors are sure to fail because your child's anxiety is not a willful act of defiance. Your equally strong desire to protect your child from the pain caused by anxiety is doomed to failure. We call this the anxiety puzzle because it is a challenging combination of problems for your whole family to solve. The solution is not a single action but hundreds of skillful acts to be performed over many years.

Although girls are more likely than boys to suffer from anxiety, plenty of boys have this problem and plenty of girls do not. Anxiety has nothing to do with being big or strong, either physically or mentally, or with intelligence, family structure, or income. Anxiety is an equal opportunity problem—it can affect anyone in any category of human existence and at any age. In this book we sometimes use the feminine pronoun to describe your child and sometimes the masculine, to reflect the fact that both boys and girls are affected.

You will learn that the only way your family can be free, kids and parents alike, is to confront anxiety every time it appears. This process of confronting fear does not have to be dramatic or Herculean. Although confronting fears can be painful to imagine, in reality the process is quite different. Rather than causing upset, confronting fears leads immediately and directly to feelings of accomplishment and to increased self-esteem. You will learn that 90 percent of the pain associated with anxiety occurs *before* the exposure to anxiety-provoking situations or experiences. Anxiety is a disorder of anticipation. It is a malignant disease of the "What if's." It is cured by the "What is's." This mystery will be explained in a later chapter of the book.

Your child can overcome anxiety problems by making gradual changes in his or her life. Persistence and patience are more important than boldness to ensure your child's long-term success. The journey to recovery is not a straight line. Long-term progress includes plenty of temporary setbacks. Because of the Dragon's great power, children and parents need real courage and determination to break free from it. You need all of the help you can get, and this includes the help of the Dragon itself, as well as that of the Wizard and the Research Notes.

## The Organization of This Book

This book is organized into three parts, a total of twelve individual chapters. Although parents and other concerned adults were our intended audience, we have made the writing accessible to child readers as well. Part One contains information about understanding children's anxiety problems.

Each of the five steps in Part Two begins with a story about a child overcoming anxiety and then details a specific, helpful step for parents. Each chapter in Part Two provides suggestions for using a Journal. You or your child will record the current state of your child's struggle with the Dragon, what parts of his life he has given up to the Dragon, and what kind of suffering the Dragon is now causing him. This is important because it documents your child's progress. From our work with victims of Dragon attacks, we have seen that unless these facts are recorded in the Journal, you and your child will quickly forget how bad things used to be. One trick the Dragon uses to keep your child in prison is the ability to make everyone forget how bad it used to be. Knowing this Dragon trick will encourage your future efforts because you'll be amazed at how far your child has come in a short period of time. You can get that perspective only by writing regularly in a Journal. It's also helpful to record specific techniques and how and when you used them.

Part Two offers concrete steps you can take to solve anxiety problems. Part Three contains important information for people in specific roles, such as teachers, or on special topics, like terrorism.

We end the book with a glossary of the language of anxiety, a listing of helpful resources, and an index.

Now you have the basic information you need to get started with *The Anxiety Cure for Kids*. Don't worry about memorizing what you read. If you are new to this subject, this book may offer too much information for you to take in all at once. The nice thing about reading a book, as opposed to visiting a therapist or a mental health professional, is that you can review the information over and over, whenever you need it. You will become familiar with these ideas as you read the book, because they are explained in great detail, along with practical advice on using them in your family's daily life.

PART ONE

*All about Anxiety*

# CHAPTER 1

# Understanding Anxiety and Fear

## *The Dragon*

This book must begin with the Dragon, because without the Dragon there is no problem. The anxiety Dragon is the cause of the disability and the distress that your child exhibits. Of course, the Dragon is an imaginary creature. Our explaining that anxiety is like a Dragon may strike some people as simplistic—or, even worse, as condescending. We see the functions of the Dragon, the Wizard, and the Research Notes quite differently. These tools are invaluable in explaining the complex biological, psychological, medical, and research components of anxiety. The field is changing rapidly, and changing for the better, as you will see in Chapter 2. For now, however, the best way to explain anxiety is to begin with the reason you picked up this book: you care about a child who is in distress. We know many children like this. Throughout the book, we give examples of kids with anxiety problems, because it is inspiring to read about other children with similar problems who got well. We have tried to keep these stories nonthreatening. We do not downplay how distressed the child was, but we also show how many options the child had, even in the tough situation in which he found himself. In this book we share with you the stories, strengths, and hopes of people who have overcome anxiety disorders.

Hello! Glad to meet you. I don't really want to hurt you or your child. I just want to protect your child—in my nice prison! It's a scary world out there. My prison is very safe.

We have taken all of the stories in this book from our many years of clinical practice. We've made changes in each story to protect the confidentiality of the families involved. To understand the power of the Dragon, you must be aware of the devastation that anxiety disorders can cause in a child's life. This book is about anxious children and the intense physical symptoms that can cause them to avoid normal activities and the pleasures of childhood. We use words like *devastating* and *intense pain* throughout the book. It is too easy for adults or people who do not have an anxiety problem themselves to underestimate the suffering that these problems can cause.

We once worked with a thirteen-year-old boy named Kurt. His parents had adopted him when he was a baby. He was African American and his parents were Caucasian. No one knew much about his biological parents, so there were no genetic clues to help anyone sort out his problems. And Kurt had problems that year. He liked to wear baggy clothes because he had gained a lot of weight over the last year when he felt bad about himself. His psychiatrist said that he was depressed. Kurt had been a worrier all his life. He also had a learning disability. That handicap made it hard for Kurt to do well in school. He had to work harder than the other students to learn things. The kids teased Kurt for being shy and worried all the time and for not being able to spell or to do math easily. Then, when Kurt gained weight, the other kids teased him even more. All Kurt really wanted to do was stay home with his mom, who loved him. He was safe at home. Kurt and his mom had fun together sometimes, but when Kurt was really sad, even being with his mom wasn't much fun. Kurt's psychiatrist helped him by having him take a medicine and then recommended that Kurt see a therapist.

Kurt was worried about seeing the therapist, especially when she asked him to keep a Journal of how he was doing. That sounded a lot like school, and right now he didn't like schoolwork. The first week Kurt didn't fill anything out in his Journal and brought it back empty. He didn't know how his therapist would react. To his surprise, she said that she had set up the Journal wrong. Instead of asking him to write in it, she wrote in it for him while they decided on goals and tasks for the week. She wrote down what Kurt told her. His words were in the Journal, but the therapist wrote them. That made it a lot easier for Kurt. She put check boxes next to the assignments so that Kurt could gauge his progress. She left a blank line for him to record, from 0 to 10, the amount of anxiety he felt during each practice session. This Kurt loved. He liked trying new ideas at school when other kids teased him. He loved having homework that asked him to play outside with a friend. After a few sessions with his therapist, Kurt felt much better. In fact, he realized that he was worrying less than he ever had in his whole life.

Kurt looked at the last assignment on the list: think about the good parts of having anxiety. When his therapist first asked him to do this, it made no sense to Kurt. What could be good about being tortured by the Dragon? It was fun finding out how to get his Wizard to fight back, but, overall, it was a lot more work and pain than not having the Dragon to begin with. Kurt spent a lot of time that week thinking about what was good about his anxiety. He thought about the boy in school who teased him the most. This mean bully had taken things from Kurt and other kids. Most of the students in Kurt's class were afraid to tell the teacher about the bully. Kurt realized that this kid had no anxiety. It didn't bother him to make other kids mad or unhappy. Kurt, on the other hand, would never steal from kids or tease them, because he knew that it would make them sad. He didn't want to hurt other children or anyone, for that matter. Kurt realized that sometimes worry was a good thing. His worry made him a better friend than if he had no worry at all. His worry made him honest. Kurt realized that some worry was a part of who he was, and that he liked that part of himself. It was great to feel that he didn't have to change a part of himself at all. He would be great, just the way he was, now that he could manage his worry.

> Anxiety is a false alarm of danger. The alarm itself is normal. The problem for your child is that his brain's alarm goes off when there is no real danger. His mind reacts to the alarm by imagining danger, which then scares him further. That false alarm of danger, repeated over and over again, causes pain, fear, and self-doubt.

This is how the Anxiety Cure works for kids. As therapists, we are lucky to see this story unfold, with endless variations, day after day. It starts out, in classic fairytale fashion, with pain and unhappiness and almost always ends with satisfaction and joy. What happens in this story may seem like magic to you, but it isn't. Though it takes hard work, the rewards are tremendous.

## Anxiety and Fear

Before you are introduced to the Dragon, the Wizard, and the Research Notes, we want to explain a few important ideas. Let's start with the word *anxiety*. It needs to be separated from *fear*. Fear is what you feel when you confront a real, immediate danger. For example, when a big bully directly threatens your daughter in the school playground, your child feels fear. When your son is climbing a tree and his feet slip out from under him, he feels fear. When your child is not facing a bully but fears going to school because a bully might be there, that is anxiety. When your child finds even looking at a tree to be scary because he might fall, that is anxiety. Fear occurs when the danger "is." Anxiety occurs when the danger "might be." Fear is generally uncommon—but familiar—in a child's life. Almost every child experiences fear in some situations. Anxiety, in clear contrast, can be a constant companion to your anxious child, in situations that would not provoke anxiety in most of your child's peers.

## Anxiety Is Made of Thoughts, Feelings, and Behaviors

*Anxiety* is a vaguely defined and commonly used word that also has a strict scientific meaning. In modern mental health research the word *anxiety* describes the thoughts, feelings, and behaviors that occur when a person has the perception of serious danger in situations where other people do not perceive danger. Anxiety means worrying that something really, really bad might happen at any minute. For example, a younger child might worry about a monster jumping out from under his bed. An older child might worry that she will be embarrassed in front of her classmates at school. For a child of any age, another serious cause of anxiety might be a major illness or the loss of a parent. Thoughts like these scare anyone. They sure can scare a child. Disturbing as these thoughts are, anxiety is more than just troubling thoughts. Strong feelings, such as tension and emotional pain, also come with anxiety. The pain can be a low-level chronic ache or a severe and acute pain. It can show up in any part of the body. Children commonly feel anxiety as a stomach ache or a headache. A person's whole body participates in the experience of anxiety, with a racing heart, tight muscles, and shallow, fast breathing. Anxiety can make a child feel that he has to urinate, defecate, or vomit.

Anxiety is even more than disturbing thoughts and painful feelings. Anxiety shows up in the anxious child's behavior. Anxiety

Over the course of a lifetime about one in every four people suffers from an anxiety disorder. Females are about twice as likely to suffer from an anxiety disorder as are males. Among children, about one in ten have an anxiety disorder. Far larger percentages of both adults and children have significant anxiety problems that do not reach the level of a "disorder." In children, anxiety problems are most likely to be seen as disruptions in normal developmental patterns. (J. March and A. M. Albano, "Anxiety Disorders in Children and Adolescents," in *Textbook of Anxiety Disorders*, 2002) causes the sufferer to pay absolute attention to the source of possible danger and to prepare to fight for his life or to immediately flee to safety. In the modern world, fighting is seldom a realistic option when anxiety makes its appearance, but flight is all too commonly the behavior that intense anxiety causes. "Get out of here right now!" "Don't go near that dangerous place!" Anxiety takes up a lot of mental capacity. Anxiety makes it hard to read or study or even to think about anything except the object of the anxiety. Anxiety is exhausting. It leads to intense fatigue and depression—to feeling defeated and helpless. These problems affect not only the child with anxiety but his entire family as well.

## The Holes Dug by Anxiety

Most anxiety-caused behaviors are children's attempts to take certain activities out of their lives. You can detect the presence of anxiety by the absence of other things, the "holes" that occur in the anxious child's life. Anxious children stick close to home and have limited social activities. There is one exception to this general rule. When children have compulsions—repetitive rituals used to ward off anxiety (such as hand-washing, for contamination fears)—then you see something abnormal added to their lives. Yet more typical of anxiety-caused behaviors is children's failure to go to school, to speak up in class, or to spend the night at a friend's house. Travel can be avoided; so can petting a dog or being in the same room with a cat. Those are important activities, the loss of which is common in the lives of anxious children. Literally thousands of abnormal holes in children's behaviors are caused by anxiety, as part of the brain's powerful automatic fight or flight response to the perception of imminent danger.

The physical and mental experience of intense worry, sometimes called a "panic attack" when it is very severe, can come out of the blue at a completely unexpected time; it's the emotional equivalent of a sudden clap of thunder on a cloudless summer day. More often, panic occurs in particular situations that are feared by the anxious child. A child with social anxiety may have panic attacks only in social settings where embarrassment is the danger, like being in a school play or even being called on to give an answer in class.

Anxiety does not always show up in a child's life as a panic attack. Anxiety can also be the low, steady rumble of a scared-to-death feeling, as if you knew there was a hungry saber-toothed tiger hiding just out of sight but ready to spring on you at any minute. Maybe that tiger is just ahead of you right now. Maybe he isn't where you think he is. You cannot be sure where he is because you don't see the tiger. Anxious children's fears tell them that the saber-toothed tiger could be almost anywhere at almost any time. Imagine trying to live a normal life with that level of fear as a menacing companion, day in and day out.

## The Good Side of Anxiety

Anxiety has a valuable biological function. Scary things do happen to children. In many situations it is good to anticipate problems because your child can then prepare for danger. That is why the capacity for anxiety is built into the human brain. Anxiety can work well to get your child's attention and to get him ready for "fight or flight" in response to real dangers. A child who is anxious about failing a test studies for the exam. A child who is anxious about a car crash wears a seat belt.

For the anxious child, this healthy brain mechanism has run amok. In most circumstances, the danger is not the saber-toothed

Anxiety disorders, in addition to being painful for the family, are also tremendously costly to society. As a class, anxiety disorders cost society $65 billion in 1994, which represents 31.8 percent of all mental health disorder costs. Though these costs are primarily caused by lost productivity in adults, the fact that most anxiety disorders originate in childhood shows that society as a whole could benefit tremendously from preventing them. (DuPont, et al., *Textbook of Anxiety Disorders*, 2002) tiger or the bully in the schoolyard but the "false alarm" itself. Nothing is there for the child to face except his own anxiety, with its associated thoughts, feelings, and behaviors. This experience of anxiety is unlike that of fear because in the child's life, it is neither rare nor brief. Pathological anxiety is often recurring and may be continuous. The problem of anxiety, however, is deeper than the false alarm because the anxious child soon comes to doubt his own body, feelings, and thoughts. He sees that other people, including children his own age, do not feel this way in this situation. Then comes an inevitable, more disturbing thought, "Something is wrong inside. Something is seriously wrong with me!" When your child has anxiety, he fears not only dangers from outside. Worse still are the terrible dangers from inside. A fearful child does not suffer from deteriorating self-esteem because the dangerous problem is *outside*. The anxious child inevitably does suffer from lowered self-esteem because the deeper, more persistent problem is clearly seen to be *inside*.

The core problem is the false alarm of danger, which produces a predictable and understandable cascade of anxious feelings, thoughts, and behaviors. The alarm is in the mid-brain, the most primitive part. It is located there because danger is such a big problem in all of life, not just in human life. The uniquely human part of the brain is the extensive cortex, the gray matter on the outside of the brain. The brain's cortex is where thinking takes place. That big cortex is the part of the brain that most makes us human. When the alarm of danger goes off, the entire cortex of the brain is put on alert. It starts working to understand and to explain the alarm, to solve the dreadful crisis that triggered the alarm in the first place. When the cortex does not immediately find a saber-toothed tiger lurking in the bushes, it uses its immense powers of imagination. That's where the "worry machine" comes into this story. In every anxious child's brain is a built-in worry machine. The worry machine harnesses the highly developed imagination that generally goes with anxiety, to spin a steady stream of stuff to worry about.

Panic happens from time to time. As the anxiety problem matures in a child, the panic typically becomes less common. In its place is worry, the "What if" syndrome of possible danger. Here is the way this works. Worry requires doubt, uncertainty. Certainty of safety is what the worried mind craves. The slightest sliver of doubt opens the floodgates of worry.

Does the worried boy know for sure that he will not get poison ivy if he goes out in that wooded area? Can he be certain that a rabid dog won't come after him if he goes outside his house? Does the anxious girl know for sure that if she goes to sleep tonight, she will wake up in the morning? Can she be sure, really, absolutely sure, that her parents will be there when she wakes up? Think of the tens of thousands of possible dire scenarios for the worry machine to work on. The worry machine is the Dragon's collaborator in the anxious child's brain. It is how the Dragon does its business, day in and day out.

---

Anxiety is genetic, in the sense that some people's brain alarms for danger are set at hair trigger and others' almost never go off, even in the scariest situations. At the same time, anxiety is environmental, in that the child's and the parent's experiences and behaviors determine what a child does about the alarm. Your child cannot change the genetic aspects of anxiety, but she can change its environmental aspects by changing her thoughts and behaviors when the alarm goes off in her brain. (U.S. Department of Health and Human Services, *Mental Health: A Report of the Surgeon General*, 1999)

---

Parents approach the problem of the anxious child's worries by reassuring the child, "Of course you won't get poison ivy, Tom, just go out with your friends and play with them." Or a parent might say, "Sally, you'll be fine tonight and when you wake up in the morning. I'll be right here." Think about it. Just how sure are those parents and how convincing are their reassurances? By now, you are saying, "But when the parent reassures the child and she comes home without poison ivy or wakes up in the morning safe and sound, then she learns to trust the parents' reassurances." Not so fast. First, many anxious children are so frightened by their worry machines that they don't do the things that they could learn from. For them, many worry scenarios are way too frightening to even try.

Besides, just because the terrible things they dread didn't happen yesterday or last night, how can they be sure these things won't happen tonight or tomorrow? If a thousand airplanes land safely, how do you know the next one will? If ten thousand planes land safely, does that guarantee the next plane will? To make the problem more realistic, think about this. Even if the anxious child does not get poison ivy or die in the night, he was very upset and in a great deal of pain as a result of the false alarm. That pain is the direct result of the magnification and elaboration of possible danger caused by the child's worry machine.

Therefore, the parents' seemingly reasonable reassurances miss the point of the child's own experience, which is terribly painful. Because other people, including the anxious child's parents, don't understand what is going on inside his mind, he feels even more alone and hopeless. The brain's false alarm starts the anxiety ball rolling. The worry machine keeps it going, day after day, month after month.

Two more points about anxiety need to be made. Anxiety is common in human experience, even where there is no saber-toothed tiger or big bully. Anxiety in some situations is even healthy and useful. For example, feeling anxious before tests at school or before acting in a school play is not only common but is usually helpful. This relatively mild anxiety encourages the child to do the homework or prepare for the part in the play. The anxiety gets the child's attention and promotes appropriate behavior. Typically, healthy anxiety is triggered over and over again in these situations and is felt by most, but not all, children. In contrast, when anxiety is associated with what most people consider normal daily activities—for example, when a child feels intense anxiety about entering an elevator because of claustrophobia, and when the anxiety is not mild but is devastatingly severe—then it is neither healthy nor useful. In this case, pathological anxiety disrupts the child's life, producing a hole (refusal to get on an elevator) in his normal behavior.

Trying hard to please others, such as friends, family, and teachers, is usually a positive characteristic that helps a reasonable person live a good life. Most anxious people automatically approach life like this. That's why anxiety is called a disease of quality people. The family team is made up of the anxious child and one or more adults—usually, but not necessarily, a parent—who work with the child daily to solve her anxiety problem. It helps to be both gentle and firm in guiding your child to confront, rather than avoid, her fears.

## Anxiety Disorders

Anxiety exists in a continuum, from mild to severe, in everyone's life. Anxiety is, however, a lot more common and intense in some people's lives than in others', even when they face similar situations. Certain situations generate more anxiety in some people than do other situations. A child who usually does well on tests is less likely to feel anxious before an exam than is a child who wants to get a good grade but has done poorly in the subject being tested. Nevertheless, most variations among children are the result of different anxiety settings in each child's brain. You probably know someone who always complains before a test that she's afraid she'll get a bad grade, yet she always gets As. After a time, her complaints become a joke. But it may not be funny if she is truly distressed, inappropriately, every time she takes a test. Some children are more prone to severe and enduring anxiety than others are. When anxiety is so severe that it leads to significant limitations in a child's life—

When panic occurs without warning, it is called "spontaneous panic." When it occurs in predictable situations (like getting on an elevator or staying overnight at a friend's house), it is called "situational panic." (*Diagnostic and Statistical Manual, IV-R*) for example, avoidance of going to school—then it is an anxiety disorder. To reach this level of a discrete mental disorder, the pathological anxiety must cause significant distress, disability, or both in the child's everyday activities.

This book was written for children whose anxiety interferes with their normal daily actions and enjoyment of life. Yet we are primarily addressing children's parents, who are their best allies in dealing with anxiety problems. We want to help, even if the child's anxiety stays below the threshold of a full-blown anxiety disorder. Because this type of anxiety is more widespread and more easily treated without professional mental health intervention or medicine, it is the primary focus of this book.

### The Dragon's Own Story

Dragons, like Wizards, do a lot of different things. Unlike other Dragons, I specialize in scaring people. You probably think I do this because I am mean. I can see why you would think that, but it is not true, or maybe I should say that it is not the whole story. I only pick on people who have false alarms of danger that ring in their heads. I don't cause that to happen; it happens all on its own. What I do is add scary thoughts to those painful feelings. I do that by magnifying and multiplying the "What if's" in the fearful person's own anxious imagination.

How do I justify myself? It's not easy, I admit, because I do cause a lot of suffering. But there is one way that I can make a claim to having a useful life. When anxious people do the work necessary to tame me, they get a huge boost in their self-esteem. They learn a wonderful technique to help them solve many of the problems they will face in their lives. So, in a way, you could call me a teacher. A harsh and an unfair teacher, that's true, but a teacher nonetheless.

I know that it's better for me and maybe it will be better for you, too, if you think of me as a teacher. At least, it gives our troublesome encounter a positive spin.

## Two Characters and One Useful Tool

You have already encountered the Dragon, the Wizard, and the Research Notes. Although you will learn more about them as you read, here are some important facts you need to know at the start. Let's start with the Dragon. It is the embodiment of anxiety and panic. When your child is anxious, he is suffering from a "Dragon attack." The Dragon is a tough beast, cruel and heartless. Like a lot of tough guys, however, it also has a tender side. If you understand it, you can tame it. The Dragon's goal is to put its victims into prison. It does this by blackmail. The Dragon comes at its victims with a dazzling show of force. It makes its victims fear the worst. It wants its victims to believe that it can make them go crazy, pass out, and lose consciousness. It wants them to believe that it can even kill them, if it chooses to. Sometimes the Dragon says it will harm or kill other people, like family members, if its victim doesn't do as it demands. This Dragon is a nasty tyrant.

There are many important things the Dragon doesn't want you and your child to know about it. For example, the only food it can eat is the fear of its victims. If they don't fear it, they don't feed it. The Dragon then withers away and withdraws from the victim's life as a result of this neglect. Its only power, really, is the power to make its victims terribly uncomfortable. It cannot do any of the awful things that it wants its victims to believe that it can do. It cannot cause physical illnesses, passing out, or loss of control. It surely cannot harm its victims, let alone kill them. The Dragon is all show and no substance, other than the pain it can inflict on its victims. That pain, however, is real. Anxiety and panic cause severe pain, as brutal as the pain of a broken leg or a heart attack. Nevertheless, knowing that the Dragon's only power is pain helps to make its attacks more endurable.

Imagine that anxiety is like a Dragon. To your child, this Dragon is huge and terrifying. It makes your child feel bad physical feelings and makes him scared. It pops up from nowhere when least expected or forces a child to perform rituals or avoid things in order to keep the Dragon away. This Dragon, of course, is all in your child's head. His own brain makes up things to be fearful of, and his mind creates panic attacks that just seem to pop up out of nowhere. Yet having the image of the Dragon is tremendously useful for both children and adults. It gives a sense of otherness to the feelings, so that they are not part of one's personality but are alien, belonging to this fierce being.

Every anxious child or adult we've ever met has instantly recognized the idea of the Dragon as appropriate for the feelings they experience. Some people call this feeling the shadow, the octopus, the beast, or the monster. We like the image of the Dragon. If your child chooses to call his anxiety a different name, just translate all of our references to the Dragon into your child's language. But first give the Dragon a try when you explain anxiety to your child. We bet that you, too, will see a light of understanding in your child's eyes.

> The first step to getting well is the most important. Your child must face the problem and accept that it is her problem to solve. She does not have to do it alone, but she has to do it. No one can do it for her, not even you, as a loving and concerned parent. The hardest thing for a parent to face is a suffering child. You want to fix your child's anxiety problem, but you cannot. Yet you can help your child fix it. Guiding you along the way is our main goal in this book.

Once the anxious child stops running away and turns to face the Dragon, the Dragon dramatically changes its behavior. It comes less often and with less intensity. But, because its attacks vary over time, it still comes back, occasionally with great force, even during your child's process of getting well. Once the child has gained control of his life, the Dragon typically goes away for short or long periods of time, sometimes for years or even decades. Sooner or later, though, the Dragon usually reappears, often with full force. At that point, the victim needs to remember the techniques for dealing with the Dragon and not flee in terror.

There is much more to know about the Dragon. It is a master of disguise. It comes at an anxious child first in one costume, then in another. That makes the Dragon hard to recognize. There is just one constant in its life: its only power is the ability to create anxiety in its victims. The Dragon's disguises are one way that it rules its victims. Sometimes it pretends to be a terrible physical illness. Sometimes it hides behind things in the environment, as if, for example, one's parents would be hurt if a child opened a door the wrong way.

> My only power is the ability to produce bad feelings. In that way I make your child afraid of what I can do to him. If your child does my bidding, I'll go a little easier on him. But I can't promise not to bother him, even if he agrees to stay in my prison. Children need constant attention. I show my attention by scaring your child.

The Dragon's goal is to put anxiety sufferers into its prison. The anxious child's goal is to be free of the Dragon. Since the child cannot directly stop the Dragon's attacks, the only way to succeed is to accept the bad feelings caused by the Dragon and to put these into a healthy perspective. That means going through life "impersonating a normal person," despite the bad feelings. When the anxious child does that, the Dragon is no longer being fed, so it soon loses interest in this particular victim. The Dragon tends to come back, but each time it returns, you can use the same techniques to limit the damage it causes.

The Research Notes of Anxiety contain the newest discoveries in the field of neuroscience, which have been pouring out of research centers around the world over the last decade. It is reassuring to know that scientists are developing better ways to understand and overcome the problems of anxiety. The Research Notes have lots of interesting, important, and practical knowledge for you and your child, and you will hear more about them in Chapter 2.

The Wizard is your guide to getting well. The Wizard is a helpful, wise, and compassionate person who understands the Dragon and who sympathizes with you and your anxious child. The Wizard offers useful ways to regain control of your anxious child's, as well as your family's, life. The Wizard knows the Dragon and all of its devious tricks and understands the information in the Research Notes. The Wizard is determined to help your anxious child stay out of the Dragon's prison. The Wizard is a guide, a pathfinder, in a world made scary by unpredictable but repeated Dragon attacks. You will read about the Wizard in Chapter 3.

The Wizard, the Dragon, and the Research Notes will provide you and your child with a shared vocabulary for thinking about anxiety and for solving this problem. Working with thousands of people—many of them children—we have found that these three tools bring the anxiety problem to life and make the solutions more understandable and practical.

*Action Steps*

- Notice the presence of the Dragon in your child's life.
- Recognize that reassuring your child does not work.
- Empathize with the suffering your child is experiencing.

# CHAPTER 2

# The History and Diagnostic Categories of Anxiety Disorders in Children and Adults

## The Language of Anxiety

In Chapter 1 you learned that severe anxiety attacks (or panic attacks) that come out of the blue are called spontaneous panic attacks, while similarly intense attacks that occur predictably in certain situations are called situational panic attacks. Spontaneous panic can be seen with all of the anxiety disorders, but it is most often seen in agoraphobia. Every anxiety disorder has two types of anxiety, the anxiety that you feel during the dreaded situation and the anxiety you feel in anticipation of the situation.

The anticipatory anxiety is far more prolonged and crippling than the anxiety felt during the painful situation itself. That is why anxiety disorders are labeled "diseases of anticipation" and "malignant diseases of the what ifs."

The intensity of anxiety disorders varies widely over the course of years. All anxiety disorders may also be lifelong in a particular person. However, the six separate anxiety disorders sometimes come and then go, leaving the previously anxious child or adult without symptoms for the rest of her life. It is impossible to predict what will happen during a lifetime. We urge you to keep hope alive that the anxiety problem may one day go away. Prudence also requires that you help your child prepare for the return of symptoms sometime in her life, even if these have been gone a long time.

In Chapter 1 we distinguished fear from anxiety. Fears are appropriate concerns about danger that is external to the child. An external danger might be a cliff at the Grand Canyon. The fear reaction is helpful because it keeps the child from falling off the edge of the cliff while hiking at the canyon. Normally, a child may be fearful of the cliff but will continue walking along the trail, knowing that if he doesn't go off the trail, he won't be in danger. Although danger is only a few inches away from the path, the path itself is safe. Most children would have the same normal, healthy fear in this or any situation with a real external danger.

Anxiety is different from fear in several important ways. First, anxiety is not shared by most of the anxious child's peers. Second, anxiety is not appropriate to the situation in which it arises. Finally, although fear does not lead to lowered self-esteem and self-doubt, anxiety usually does. With children the separation of fear from anxiety can be more challenging than it is with adults. Children often have age-appropriate fears that in a child of a different age are no longer age appropriate and are described as anxiety. For example, fears that cause children to cling to parents and be reluctant to go to school are common during the first few grades. Usually brief and quickly overcome, these are considered age-appropriate fears. The same behavior in older children would be identified as anxiety, because it is no longer age-appropriate.

Similarly, many early adolescent children are socially insecure. Social fears at this age are considered age-appropriate if they are relatively brief, don't interfere with the child's development, and are similar to fears felt by the child's peers. Any fear that dominates a child's life, limits his daily experience, or persists over a long period of time is probably anxiety.

One more term needs to be defined in regard to children's anxiety problems: the word *phobia*. A phobia is a fear of a particular object or experience that leads to anxious avoidance. A child with a phobia of dogs, for example, may be so upset by anxious feelings that even the thought of a dog makes her not want to leave home. She may refuse to visit a friend's house just because the friend or the friend's neighbor has a dog. The hallmark of phobia is avoiding a situation or an experience that most of one's peers do not avoid. Phobias tend to be highly focused and specific, while anxiety is more diffuse, more generalized, and less limited to a single object or experience. A wide variety of phobias often accompanies anxiety disorders in children, including fears of the dark and of monsters, kidnappers, bugs, small animals, heights, and both open and enclosed spaces. Resistance to going to sleep at night or to sleeping through the night, especially when alone, and nightmares with separation themes are common in anxious children. In assessing a child for anxiety problems, you should carefully note problem behaviors, such as phobic avoidance, and get the child's own description of her feelings and thoughts. Without the child's self-report of her inner experiences, the anxiety problem may remain hidden from adults.

Two more key words must be added to your anxiety vocabulary. The first is *alone*. All of the anxiety disorders lead sufferers to doubt themselves, to feel cut off from others, and, ultimately, to feel alone with their anxiety, intense pressure, pain, and suffering. When you feel alone, you feel vulnerable and even helpless.

The second word in your new anxiety vocabulary is *trapped*. All of the anxiety disorders have, at their root, claustrophobia. The sufferer feels trapped with the anxiety problem. He feels he cannot shake it, no matter how hard he tries to bargain with the blackmailing Dragon. He cannot get away from the dreadful feelings of anxiety. He is trapped in his own mind by the pain of anxiety. He also feels trapped in his life, surrounded by triggers to situational panic. The person with elevator phobia is surrounded—trapped— by elevators. She never knows when she'll need to get into an elevator. One girl felt crippled, day in and day out, by the thought that she might get sick and need to be hospitalized, "and you know that hospitals are full of elevators." Thus, even if she had not seen an elevator for weeks or months, elevators were a threat to her every single minute.

These words—*alone* and *trapped*—are vital to understanding and communicating with your anxious child. You need to help your child learn that "alone" and "trapped" are states of thinking, not states of being. No one is ever truly alone. No one is ever truly trapped. People who can help are always around. There are always escape routes. We will teach you more about how to deal with these universal anxious thoughts, which are such an obstacle to your child's progress.

> The core fear in agoraphobia is not of the market but of the panic feelings of being trapped away from a safe person or a safe place. These feelings are feared understandably but unreasonably.

## Anxious Feelings Are Real and Severe

As you think about your child's anxiety problem, we need to dispel one dangerous misunderstanding. Everyone has anxiety. This fact makes it easy for people without anxiety problems to compare their own anxieties to the experiences of people suffering from significant, pathological anxiety. In this misguided view, people without an anxiety problem are emotionally "strong" and those with an anxiety problem are emotionally "weak." The error here is in not realizing that these experiences of anxiety are not only different in degree but different in kind.

The person suffering with an anxiety problem has very uncomfortable feelings. In addition, many people with anxiety develop beliefs that the danger alarm going off in their brains must reflect real external danger, even though they know that others do not perceive danger in similar situations. The person who fears being trapped in an elevator knows that other people don't fear elevators; nevertheless, she believes that she will be trapped and unable to breathe in a stuck elevator. Over time, this pattern of pathological anxiety intensifies, separating the anxious person from those who don't have anxiety problems. Don't assume that your anxiety is like your anxious child's experience unless you also suffer from a serious anxiety problem. Making that assumption will undermine your ability to help your child. He will think that you don't understand his experience and that you see him as weak or inadequate.

Recent research has shown that anxiety disorders are the most common mental disorders in children, with about one in eight children being affected. This is more than twice the rate for mood disorders, including depression and bipolar disorder. Anxiety disorders, overall, are more common in girls than in boys. Children with a parent who has an anxiety disorder are more than three times as likely to have this problem themselves, as are those children whose parents did not have an anxiety disorder.

Anxiety shows as feelings, thoughts, and behaviors related to the threat of danger, even though this external danger is small or nonexistent. The anticipated danger is not outside of the anxious child, it is inside. This internal anxiety is in contrast to the Grand Canyon example of external fear. Internal anxiety is a truly painful feeling. The anticipation of experiencing this painful feeling produces upsetting thoughts and avoidant behaviors. Anxiety is the brain's healthy, useful alarm signaling danger when there is no realistic external threat. Anxiety is a false alarm in your child's nervous system. It is real, serious, and painful. It is especially disturbing to a child who lacks an adult understanding of anxiety problems. Anxiety in children is usually seen in behaviors that reflect fear and the need for protection, reassurance, and escape.

Anxiety problems show up as holes in the child's life. The child avoids certain things because he fears the bad feelings that anxiety produces. At relatively low levels and in appropriate situations, anxiety can be useful to a child, but if it is severe and occurs when no real external danger is present, it isn't helpful. Feeling a low level of

Anxious people are good people who are suffering from a bad problem. Working hard to overcome anxiety problems can become a big source of self-esteem and self-respect.

anxiety in anticipation of a test at school is healthy. Yet a high level of anxiety may make it impossible for a child to take the test or even go to school that day. This is not healthy; it is likely to be an anxiety problem.

Anxious adults, as well as anxious children, realize that their feelings are unusual, so they often hide the reasons they don't do things, to escape people's criticism. Even so, adults commonly put their feelings of anxiety into words. Children are less likely than adults to say, "I'm anxious" or "I'm worried" and are more likely to act out their anxiety by changing their behavior—for example, by not going to school or not staying overnight with a friend. Children are more likely than adults to show anxiety by complaining about illness, especially headaches and stomach aches, because they quickly learn that physical problems can help them avoid situations that may produce anxiety, like going to school or taking a test.

You know your child has an anxiety problem when you see maladaptive behaviors—usually, avoidance behaviors that are the result of the "flight" aspect of the fight-or-flight response to impending perceived dangers. Clinging to adults, especially parents, and refusing to go to new or unfamiliar places are common signs of anxiety in younger children. Older anxious children are more likely to hide their anxiety by simply saying, "I don't want to do it," when faced with things that make them anxious. Sometimes older children engage in disruptive behavior to get out of things they don't want to do. This is not common among anxious adolescents, though, because they are usually scrupulous about avoiding criticism from adults in authority, such as parents and teachers.

> Encourage your child to become a student of her anxiety and learn what makes it go up and what makes it go down. Your child will feel less anxious when she can touch someone, and when she talks about her feelings and thoughts. These connections with others reduce feelings of being trapped and alone.

As a parent, you want your child to take full advantage of the abundant opportunities that life offers. When your anxious child pulls back from ordinary life experiences, this is a sign that he may have an anxiety problem. Although anxiety is unitary, the behaviors that show anxiety vary and so do the triggers of anxiety for individual children. What makes one anxious child terribly upset will be no problem whatsoever for another anxious child. Specific anxiety-triggering situations and behavioral responses to these create a particular anxious child's patterns of anxiety. These destructive patterns are reflected in the six core anxiety disorders, which are described later in this chapter. Although this book is meant for children who have anxiety problems but don't necessarily suffer from anxiety disorders, nevertheless, it's helpful for parents to understand the six specific anxiety disorders. In this way, the child's anxiety problems can be characterized and parents can think more clearly about what needs to be done. Of all the mental disorders of childhood, anxiety disorders are usually the first to appear. Children who have untreated anxiety disorders are more likely to have a variety of other problems, often later in their lives—with depression during young adulthood being particularly common.

## The Historical Categories of Childhood Anxiety

To understand the modern categories of anxiety disorders, it's useful to have a historical overview. For decades, child psychiatry was a separate medical specialty, with its own language and diagnostic categories. Child psychiatrists were usually psychoanalysts who specialized in using play therapy to work with children, much in the style of Anna Freud, Sigmund Freud's brilliant daughter. The goal of child therapy was to identify and then work through the unconscious conflicts that led to the child's psychopathology. Sigmund Freud considered anxiety the result of repressed thoughts and wishes. In his later years, Freud thought of anxiety as having two major sources: the first was being overwhelmed by sexual or aggressive stimulation, and the second was the anticipation of danger, which produced signal anxiety, a warning of imminent harm. The anxious person mobilized "defenses" against threatening instinctual excitation. The specific defenses that were mobilized produced the distinctive patterns of anxiety problems in adults and children.

Parents, especially mothers, often were seen as the source of the child's anxiety problems. Anxiety was the core mental problem in the psychoanalytic perspective on childhood, as well as in adult mental disorders. The specific pathological behaviors of the child were seen as strategies the child used to ward off anxiety. Anxiety in childhood was separated into three separate categories or diagnoses: separation anxiety disorder, avoidance disorder of childhood or adolescence, and overanxious disorder. In this early era of child psychiatry, medications were seldom used.

## The New View of Anxiety in Children

These three separate diagnoses for childhood anxiety were established when psychoanalysis was dominant in American psychiatry, for adults as well as for children, and when the anxiety disorders were generally thought to be trivial, rare, and hopeless. These attitudes began to change in the late 1970s, when there was a new focus on adult anxiety disorders. This new focus can be traced to three major developments. First, a new manual was developed in 1980, the *Diagnostic and Statistical Manual of Mental Disorders-Third Edition* (*DSM-III*), which was based not on psychoanalytic theories of mental disorders but on a description of the symptoms experienced by psychiatric patients. This new set of diagnoses grouped the anxiety disorders according to the common patterns of the most prominent anxiety symptoms. The second new development in the 1980s was the application of these more objectively defined diagnoses to large samples of the U.S. population. New epidemiological studies produced the first-ever estimates of the extent to which specific mental disorders were found in the nation. To the surprise of mental health experts, anxiety disorders were the most common group of all the mental health disorders, exceeding, for example, both depression and schizophrenia. This same study showed that anxiety disorders produced more disability and a higher overall social burden than did any other group of mental disorders.

The third new development in the modern understanding of anxiety also occurred in the 1980s, with the demonstration that anxiety disorders responded favorably to both cognitive-behavioral treatment (CBT) and to medications, especially to antidepressants. These developments, taken together, revolutionized modern medicine's thinking about anxiety disorders. At the end of the twentieth century they were shown to be not trivial, not rare, and not hopeless. The use of medications got a huge boost with the new generation of antidepressants, starting with Prozac, Zoloft, and Paxil, all of which had powerful beneficial effects on anxiety disorders, whether the anxious patient also had depression or not. These developments revolutionized thinking and opened up a far more hopeful era for people suffering from anxiety problems.

Prior to this time, anxiety disorders were rarely diagnosed and poorly understood, even by mental health professionals. They were seldom treated successfully. During the last two decades, anxiety disorders have rivaled depression as the subject of professional and popular attention. Newspapers, magazines, television, and the Internet now have an abundance of information about anxiety disorders. People don't have to rely on mental health professionals for the latest scientific discoveries. The mass media have recognized the widespread extent of anxiety problems and are sure to highlight any news on the subject. They do this not only as a public service but also in their own self-interest because a huge audience exists for these reports.

The one-word antidote for all anxiety problems is *acceptance*. This starts with acceptance of the painful feelings of panic and anxiety. Acceptance is the opposite of avoiding your fears. Avoidance cannot be tolerated if your child is going to get well.

## Anxiety in Children and Adolescents

Initially, these dramatic new developments focused exclusively on adults with anxiety disorders. Although children with anxiety were left out of this first wave of interest, the winds of change stirred through the field of child psychiatry during the 1990s. The use of Ritalin and other stimulants to treat attention deficit hyperactivity disorder (ADHD) brought medications into child psychiatry in a big way. The public became aware of ADHD, as the use of medications to treat it was hotly debated. More directly, the initial epidemiological studies of mental disorders had population samples that began at age eighteen. Although children were not included in these study samples, researchers soon found that anxiety disorders rates were already high by age eighteen. Furthermore, they found that symptoms of adult anxiety disorders usually began in childhood, often at a very young age. A few mental health pioneers began to use CBT and antianxiety medications to treat children with anxiety disorders. These modern treatments, which had recently become common for adults with anxiety problems, were soon found to have equally good results in children.

Many studies have confirmed that among children and adolescents, anxiety disorders are the most common of all mental health problems. The rate of anxiety disorders in children is believed to be between 6 percent and 10 percent, nationally. This high rate has spurred interest in studies to determine which methods are most effective in preventing and treating anxiety problems in children. (McCracken, et al. *Journal of Clinical Psychiatry*, vol. 63, suppl. 6 [2002]: 8–11)

Beginning in 1994, the diagnostic labels of specific adult anxiety disorders were applied to children's disorders, ending a decade of using unique psychoanalytic labels for children with anxiety. This development signaled the recognition that each individual anxiety disorder extended over the human life cycle and often began in childhood. This, coupled with the realization that the same treatments that were effective for adults were also effective for children, inaugurated the twenty-first-century focus on anxiety disorders in children. The pharmaceutical companies, which had pioneered the use of antidepressants to treat anxiety disorders in adults—even in the absence of depression—competed with each other to win FDA (U.S. Food and Drug Administration) approval of their medications to treat anxiety disorders in childhood. This flood of interest encouraged more fundamental research in the early development of anxiety problems.

> Modern medicines put a muzzle on me. They make it harder for me to scare the daylights out of your child because your child's brain doesn't produce so many false alarms of danger once the medicines have had time to work.

Twenty, even ten years ago, anxiety disorders were rarely diagnosed, even in adults. Childhood anxiety was widely seen as either a stage the child would outgrow or as an insignificant problem of temperament. As anxiety disorders have taken center stage with both the public and mental health professionals, there has been a shift from greatly underdiagnosing anxiety in children to sometimes overdiagnosing it. This is because more people now understand and recognize anxiety as both common and treatable. Rather than being one of the last diagnoses to be considered, anxiety disorders are now one of the first. The reality is that anxiety is often seen in virtually all mental disorders—not just anxiety disorders but mood disorders such as major depression and bipolar disorder. Anxiety is also common in substance-use disorders, conduct disorders, and even psychotic disorders, such as schizophrenia. All of these conditions have anxiety as a prominent symptom. It wasn't by accident that Sigmund Freud, more than a hundred years ago, put anxiety at the center of mental life, as well as at the center of mental disorders.

Children who are especially fearful of the physical feelings of anxiety (heart beating fast, sweaty palms, feeling dizzy, upset stomach, etc.) are more prone to develop panic disorder. They are not more likely to develop the other anxiety disorders. (Chorpita, *Journal of Abnormal Child Psychology*, vol. 30, no. 2 [April 2002]: 177–90)

If your child has pervasive and serious behavioral problems, beyond simple anxiety, it is wise to get the opinion of a trained mental health professional before you assume that your child's problem is primarily, or only, an anxiety problem. As you read this book, think about whether your child's problems fit within the patterns that we describe.

One more caution needs to be added. Worry is the hallmark of anxiety and parents of anxious children often have heightened anxiety themselves. If we describe any problem, however uncommon it may be, anxious parents reading this book are likely to apply it to themselves and their children. Part of the worry disease is to perceive trouble even when it isn't there. Ten readers of this book—no, make that one hundred readers—will falsely assume that their child's anxiety problem is something more serious than an anxiety disorder, for every one parent who errs in the opposite direction and assumes that her child has an anxiety problem when it is actually some other, less easily treated mental disorder, such as schizophrenia.

## Anxiety in Children—The Goal Is Prevention

One other development was vital to the emerging priority given to anxiety in children. School-based programs in New Zealand fostered hope that if anxiety problems were dealt with more effectively in childhood, fewer children would develop full-blown anxiety disorders. In addition, even if some anxious children did, as adults their symptoms would be less and the disability caused by their anxiety would be eliminated entirely. In summary, the modern era of focus on childhood anxiety disorders had at least three sources: first, the recognition that anxiety disorders usually begin in childhood; second, that childhood anxiety disorders respond to the same medical and nonmedical treatments that adult disorders do; and third, that if anxiety is well treated in childhood, this could prevent the later emergence of adult anxiety disorders.

> One of my best strategies is to make your child afraid of embarrassment. This strategy works especially well with teenagers.

## The Six Anxiety Disorders

As you deal with your child's anxiety, it's useful to keep in mind the six major categories of anxiety disorders. To rise to the level of a diagnosable mental disorder, the anxiety problem must have persisted for at least six months, it cannot be caused by some other medical or psychiatric problem (such as depression or illicit drug use), and it must significantly interfere with the person's life, cause a great degree of distress, or both.

> There are six separate anxiety disorders, but worry is the common element in all of them.

Look at each diagnosis in turn, to see how it shows up in children and adults. This book contains examples of children with various anxiety diagnoses. As you think about your child's symptoms, take a look at these stories to clarify how the different anxiety problems manifest. Chapter 8, about school anxiety, gives examples of how each diagnostic category can cause a multitude of school problems. We provide specific types of Wizard magic for the school setting.

| DSM-IV Category | Story of a Child with This Problem | Typical Symptoms in Children |
| --- | --- | --- |
| Panic Disorder/ Agoraphobia | Ben, Chapter 5 Rebecca, Chapter 8 Joseph, Chapter 8 | Fear of having a spontaneous or situational panic attack, often along with a fear of being away from home or away from a safe person. |
| Social Anxiety Disorder (SAD) | Jenny, Chapter 8 | Severe shyness; fear of talking in a group or in class; fear of parties; fear of public speaking. |
| Obsessive-Compulsive Disorder (OCD) | William, Chapter 7 | Severe obsessions causing the performance of rituals, such as hand washing or checking. |
| Generalized Anxiety Disorder (GAD) | Kurt, Chapter 1 Ryan, Chapter 8 | Severe, almost continuous, inappropriate worry about many topics. |
| Specific Phobic Disorder | Julie, Chapter 6 Tanya, Chapter 8 | Phobia of cats, dogs, or other animals or bugs; fear of heights; fear of the dark. |
| Posttraumatic Stress Disorder (PTSD) | Morgan, Chapter 8 | Severe anxiety that occurs after an extreme trauma; may feel like the trauma is continuing. |

## Panic Disorder/Agoraphobia

Panic disorder/agoraphobia was the first anxiety disorder to gain widespread public and professional attention in the 1980s. Many people think of it as causing the most suffering and disability. Panic disorder is diagnosed when a person has repeated, severe, spontaneous panic attacks that are painful and crippling. Agoraphobia is avoidance that is based on the fear of being away from a safe person or a safe place. The Greek term *agora* means "marketplace." *Phobia* means avoidance based on fear of a specific situation or experience. Literally, agoraphobia means "fearful avoidance of the marketplace." The syndrome got this name because sufferers, who were normal in other ways, were afraid to leave home and go out to the market. Although their problem was not the market, but leaving home, early observers didn't make this connection and misapplied the diagnostic term. This syndrome would have been more accurately called "fear of leaving the safety of home."

The modern understanding of agoraphobia is that the fear is not only of being away from home but of being away from familiar places. Agoraphobia is also the fear of being alone. The person suffering from agoraphobia typically feels anticipatory anxiety when even thinking of leaving home or being alone. The anxiety symptoms are lessened when the sufferer is with a trusted, familiar person. It isn't hard to see the connection of this syndrome to children's fear of being away from home or from their parents and siblings. These children feel reassured when their parents, especially their mothers, accompany them into unfamiliar places. Thus the syndrome of agoraphobia is often labeled "separation anxiety." When seen in adults, where it is common, agoraphobia is best thought of as "adult separation anxiety." It is possible to suffer from panic disorder without also having agoraphobia. Usually, the problem begins with panic disorder and then, over time, the sufferer anticipates future panic attacks, which are understandably but erroneously thought to be life-threatening. Soon, the panic sufferer seeks the safety and security of familiar places and reliable people, just in case the panic strikes again.

Agoraphobia can also exist without panic attacks, although this is not common. When it occurs, this often reflects long-standing agoraphobia. In these cases, the panic has usually long since faded away, leaving only the agoraphobia. Typically, panic attacks precede the emergence of the agoraphobia.

People who are unfamiliar with the disorder naturally assume that someone who has agoraphobia is "weak," "immature," "dependent," or even "childlike." Although this may be true for some people, many children and adults—men and women alike—who suffer from agoraphobia are remarkably strong and mature. How can that be? Why, then, do they show early childhood symptoms of separation anxiety? That is where panic disorder comes into the picture. The agoraphobia sufferer typically fears not the marketplace but the panic attack. Panic often comes when the person feels trapped or alone. The sufferer is crippled by the fear and anticipation of a panic attack that may come at any time. The most prominent feature of agoraphobia, and of all anxiety disorders, is anticipatory anxiety. Because the agoraphobia sufferer believes that the panic will produce not just unpleasant feelings but loss of control, going crazy, or even sudden death, he works hard to avoid situations that could trigger a panic attack. Since panic attacks cannot be completely avoided, the agoraphobic wants to be with someone who can call for help if necessary and wants to stay in safe, familiar places in case panic strikes out of the blue. That's how a person suffering from panic attacks gets agoraphobia. Agoraphobia is the understandable reaction to the fear of life-threatening and terribly painful panic attacks.

## Social Anxiety Disorder (SAD)

Social anxiety disorder (SAD; formerly called social phobia) is different from agoraphobia in one striking way. Being with other people—rather than being alone—triggers the panic. In fact, many people with social anxiety disorder are more comfortable being alone than they are with others. They feel especially upset when in the presence of an unfamiliar person or an authority figure who might criticize them. The person's core fear is of embarrassment. This typically leads to avoidance of social encounters, especially with people who are not well known, because strangers can't be trusted not to embarrass the person who has social anxiety disorder. This avoidance can lead to failure to make friends and to restricted social activities. People with SAD may fear giving a speech, speaking up in class, or even meeting or talking with strangers or people in authority, because these situations might embarrass them.

Social anxiety disorder comes in two forms. The generalized form of SAD is an extreme form of shyness, a crippling shyness. Many or perhaps all unfamiliar people are feared as a source of potential embarrassment. Often, the person with SAD fears sweating or blushing, which would call attention to himself. In the specific form of SAD, as contrasted with generalized SAD, the fear of embarrassment is limited to public speaking or presentations. This specific anxiety can become so intense that it is hard or almost impossible to speak up in class or at a meeting, even just to say your name aloud to a group.

SAD leads to avoidance of social encounters, which can be extremely crippling to children in school and to adults later in life. For example, many young people with SAD stop their schooling to avoid embarrassment in class. At work, people with SAD not only fail to give presentations and speeches, they often leave jobs because they might be called upon to speak in small groups.

## Obsessive-Compulsive Disorder (OCD)

Obsessive-compulsive disorder is a different sort of anxiety problem. Obsessions are unwanted, unpleasant thoughts that get stuck in the anxious person's head. An example is the worry "If I touch that door handle, my mother will die," or "If I eat that particular food, I'll get cancer." These alarming thoughts would disturb anyone. For most of us, thoughts like this are fleeting and quickly dismissed as unreasonable, although they do make us uncomfortable when they occur. For a person with OCD, these thoughts are constant companions. The repugnant thoughts get stuck in the sufferer's head, like a record that plays the same musical phrase over and over and over again. These repetitive, disturbing thoughts are the way the anxiety Dragon does its work. The foreign thoughts lead to intense anxiety, which can be reduced only by the "compulsions." These are ritualized, mindless activities that alleviate the anxiety produced by the obsessions. Examples of compulsions are not touching particular doors or else ritualized or magical door touching (three times or thirty times in a precise way), avoidance of certain foods, or excessive hand washing to avoid contamination. In the other five anxiety disorders, what we see is what is missing from the sufferer's life. With OCD, we see what is added—for example, touching the door in bizarre ways. Because the sufferer knows this behavior is incomprehensible, he often conceals the compulsive act so that other people, including his parents, don't notice it.

Sometimes obsessions are scary because the sufferer fears that he will harm someone else. For example, even the sight or the thought of a knife can be scary because the person with OCD fears that he will stab someone he loves. This is an obsession when it gets stuck in the anxious person's mind or when it returns over and over again. Commonly, this obsession leads to the compulsive avoidance of knives or scissors, to avoid the possibility of impulsively grabbing one of these instruments. We, personally, have never seen (or even heard of) a person with OCD actually stabbing someone. We remind sufferers with OCD that they cannot control their thoughts and feelings, but they can control their behavior. They need to let those nasty obsessional thoughts go and not add fearful thoughts to them. OCD thoughts are always repulsive, upsetting, and contrary to the sufferer's own character.

Children may go through a developmentally normal stage of superstition that looks like OCD. A common example is a child who doesn't want to step on a crack after hearing the rhyme "Step on a crack and break your mother's back." In most cases, this type of superstition is short-lived and doesn't cause significant disability. A similar, developmentally normal pattern occurs when some early teens begin to keep themselves fastidiously clean. Parents may complain that a child changes outfits several times a day and wants clothes washed after only a few hours of wear. It's important to evaluate the duration of the problem, the disability caused by it, and the degree of suffering the child experiences. Typically, a child who doesn't have OCD but just normal developmental hyper-

THE HISTORY AND DIAGNOSTIC CATEGORIES

caution about cleanliness will help with laundry or stop changing clothes so often when a parent points out the unreasonableness of this behavior. Even if the teen protests or complains, he will continue to lead his life normally, while adjusting to a change in the way he dresses and grooms himself. In contrast, a child with OCD will show tremendous distress, perhaps even becoming nonfunctional, if a parent places "contaminated" clothing with "clean" clothing. In OCD not only is the behavior severe, it persists despite parental and other interventions.

 Fear is a weak tool for me, but anxiety will cut the legs out from under anyone. I can get people, even very strong people, into my prison with the power of anxiety.

## Generalized Anxiety Disorder (GAD)

Generalized anxiety disorder is the foundation of all anxiety problems. It consists of worry and tension without the distinctive features that characterize the other five anxiety disorders. Many people with GAD occasionally experience symptoms of other anxiety disorders, but their enduring experience is of generalized anxiety that waxes and wanes over their entire lives. With GAD, in contrast to phobias, the source of the worry is spread among many experiences and threats. It is not focused on any one object or experience. Children with GAD seem to be "born worriers" who worry about many things. For example, they may worry about school, health, a parent's safety, or anything and everything. GAD comes from the worry machine in a child's mind, churning out a malicious flood of "what ifs," one worry after another, endlessly.

## Specific Phobic Disorder

Specific phobic disorder is the classic one-cause phobia, such as fear of dogs or spiders, claustrophobia, or fear of flying, without the other features of agoraphobia or panic disorder. When you see multiple phobias, it is usually from agoraphobia, not from a specific phobic disorder. Like GAD, specific phobic disorder is a diagnosis of exclusion. This means that if a person has claustrophobia or another specific phobia *and* a social anxiety problem or a panic problem, then the diagnosis is not specific phobic disorder, but the other condition, such as agoraphobia or social anxiety disorder. If people with specific phobias also suffer from worry and anxiety, not just worry related to the object of their specific phobia (for example, if they are afraid of dogs and they worry excessively about lots of other things as well), they are diagnosed with GAD and not with specific phobic disorder.

## Posttraumatic Stress Disorder (PTSD)

Most people have stressful experiences in their lives that suddenly produce an increase in anxiety. The diagnosis of PTSD is reserved for people who have truly unusual and extreme traumas, such as seeing someone murdered before their eyes or being in a dreadful automobile accident in which they are seriously injured or someone close to them is hurt or killed. Rape, assault, and war are all examples of extreme traumas. In response to these stresses, the PTSD sufferer has flashbacks and nightmares of the traumatic event. Anxiety, as well as depression, is a prominent and enduring feature of PTSD. Many people feel anxiety after extreme stress, but their symptoms fade over the course of weeks or months, and the anxiety doesn't interfere with their lives. For PTSD to be diagnosed, the anxiety symptoms must persist for at least six months after the stressful event and must produce significant disruption in the sufferer's life. Most soldiers who survive a terrible battle don't suffer from PTSD. The question of who will develop PTSD after a trauma is still being researched, but we do know that the vulnerability of the sufferer relates not only to the trauma itself but also to the brain's specific reaction to the trauma.

## Scoring Your Child's Anxiety

Anxiety varies over the course of months, years, and even decades; it also changes over very short periods of time, such as seconds or minutes. One minute your child's anxiety can be severe and the next minute only mild or even nonexistent. It's important for you and your child to study his anxiety. Rate the level of your child's anxiety from 0, for none at all, to 10, for the worst panic attack that he has ever had. Talk with him about the precise level of anxiety he feels at each minute and over the course of weeks or months. This is a big part of controlling the anxiety problem. Study together what makes the level of anxiety go up and what makes it go down. Remember, no matter how high the level of anxiety gets, it will go down. Even the greatest anxiety usually dissipates quickly. Part Two of this book offers specific advice on keeping track of your child's anxiety.

Even when you aren't using the Wizard's magic and the Research Notes, it's important to score your child's anxiety, because the Dragon wants you and your child to believe that his anxiety goes just one way—up, up, and up. Talk with your child about how and when the anxiety goes down and what you both can do to get it down. Just defining your child's problem as anxiety helps bring his anxiety levels down. What increases your child's anxiety is fearing the rising level of anxiety. Your child's fear is feeding the Dragon! The more he fears his rising feelings of anxiety, the more his anxiety will rise.

> I just figured out that if you and your child both work on your anxiety problems, you both will escape from my prison! That's not what I have in mind for the two of you.

Panic disorder/agoraphobia, generalized anxiety disorder, and specific phobic disorder are each about twice as common in females as in males. The same ratio is true for depression, which is also about twice as common in females as in males. In contrast, obsessive-compulsive disorder, social anxiety disorder, and post-traumatic stress disorder are about equally common in males and females. No one knows why these ratios apply, but it is thought that they reflect both biological and cultural factors.

Each anxiety disorder can occur with any of the other anxiety disorders. A person with agoraphobia may also have social anxiety disorder. All of the anxiety disorders are commonly seen with depression. The usual convention is to label the most troubling or crippling anxiety disorder the primary diagnosis and others that occur in a particular person the secondary diagnoses. Another way to determine the primary diagnosis is to identify which problem came first. For example, it's common for an anxiety disorder to start in childhood and depression to begin in young adulthood. In that case, the anxiety disorder may be considered as primary because it began first.

In this chapter we reviewed the six major anxiety disorders because they define the common patterns of anxiety problems, even if those problems do not reach the level of a specific mental disorder. When anxiety doesn't rise to this level, it's called "sub-syndromal." Far more people suffer from subsyndromal anxiety problems than suffer from anxiety disorders. This is especially true for children.

---

Anxiety disorders seldom come alone in children. They are often hooked up with other mental health problems, most frequently with depression. In children, there is a strong link between having a generally negative outlook in life and being likely to have anxiety, depression, or both. Having a positive outlook predicts that children may have anxiety, but it is not usually linked to depression. (Chorpita, *Journal of Abnormal Child Psychology*, vol. 30, no. 2 (April 2002): 177–90)

We don't expect you to become an expert mental health diag-
nostician, but recognizing your anxious child's problems will help
you understand the patterns of clinically significant anxiety. Anxiety problems, like anxiety disorders, are commonly seen in these six
patterns. Your new understanding will help you find the self-help
literature on the topic of your child's specific anxiety problem. You
will be able to talk about her problem with experts, including people at her school, pediatricians, and mental health professionals.
Remember, though—as helpful as diagnostic labels are, it's important not to let labels get in the way of observing your child's specific
problems. So, when you talk to others about her anxiety, don't rely
only on the diagnostic label but also describe the specific behaviors
or feelings that your child experiences.

*Action Steps*

- Write down the category or categories of anxiety that seem
  most closely to fit your child's problem.
- Evaluate how your child's anxiety is different from or similar
  to that of his peers.

# CHAPTER 3

# Treatment
## *The Wizard*

The Dragon causes anxiety symptoms, but the Wizard helps you to help your child. Even better, your child herself can learn to use the calm, rational tone of the Wizard. The more she fears the feelings that the anxiety Dragon gives her, the more the Dragon grows. These feelings are tremendously distressing, but *they are not dangerous*. It is easy for you, as a parent, to get pulled into trying to reassure your child that what she fears is not worthy of fear. The problem is that this gives the Dragon power by allowing the false, anxiety-caused topic to remain an essential part of the conversation. The real topic is the fear of the feeling, not whatever the Dragon causes a child to fear.

This cannot be stated often enough. The fear, not the situation, is the problem. This is the Wizard's most important message and one that can be extremely hard to understand. It seems like the problem is the specific situation—after all, that's what your child tells you. Parents are an essential first line of defense in helping a child change her outlook and recognize a Dragon attack for what it is. Over time, it's important for the child herself to learn the Wizard's voice, but, initially, parents almost always have to play a role in helping the child learn this new way of thinking.

## The Wizard's Own Story

I didn't start out wanting to be a Wizard. Many years ago, before anyone knew much about anxiety, I was a scientist trying to earn a Ph.D. in the study of insect biology. Without warning, when I was about twenty-five, I had a terrible panic attack. I thought that I was going to die right then. Doctors and their medicines could not help me. Neither could my teachers or my parents. I quit my university studies and took to bed. I waited to die, as I suffered through one panic attack after another. My uncle, who lived in another city, came to visit me. A doctor who had served in the First World War, he had seen many cases of "shell shock." That's what doctors called posttraumatic stress disorder at that time. He said he had learned that soldiers with shell shock were better off if they went back to the front right away, rather than staying in hospitals. He advised me to do that—to get out of my bed and go back to the university, no matter how many panic attacks I had. He said that the panic could not hurt me physically—let alone kill me.

I followed his advice. Over time and with a lot of effort, it worked. At that point, I decided that I wanted to help other people with this dreadful problem. It was clear to me that most doctors and other health-care workers did not understand the problem or how to help young people with panic and anxiety. Six years later I got my degree in Wizardry. Ever since, I have worked with doctors and scientists, and especially with anxious children and their parents, to solve the crippling and painful problem of pathological anxiety. I've had a wonderfully satisfying career and have helped a lot of young people and their families. I've learned a lot about that Dragon, most of which it didn't want me to know.

Wizard magic works best if you and your child think through this new way of looking at the problem at a time when the Dragon is not attacking. When your child is at a high level of anxiety, it's tough for him to learn this new skill. But after you both have discussed the problems that the Dragon is causing him, you will both be able to identify the problem even when your child is in a high state of anxiety.

> The Dragon doesn't want you to know that the only food it can eat is your fear. Stop fearing it and that scary Dragon will wither away.

One of our patients was a ten-year-old boy who had obsessive-compulsive disorder. At a family Fourth of July party, there were several piñatas filled with candy. The boy became worried that a candy wrapper paper was stuck to his teeth. He was so fearful that it might cause him to choke and die, he couldn't enjoy the party. He made his mom miserable, too, asking for reassurance over and over again. She was pulled into his distress.

Using a standard scale to rate anxiety—from 0, representing no anxiety, to 10, which is the worst anxiety a person ever experienced—is another helpful Wizard tool. This language improves communication immensely, especially in tough moments. Without the language of anxiety rating, a kid has to show you how bad a situation is by being loud, crying, or otherwise demonstrating distress. With this 0 to 10 scale, a child can immediately convey his feelings. Acting out his distress and using inflammatory language would tend to make the kid feel even more out of control. Since this boy and his mother had already been working with a Journal and keeping track of anxiety levels for a few weeks, he could clearly tell his mom he was at Level 8 with his anxiety.

> One of my best tricks is to make a kid focus on some small thing that isn't quite right. Then I tell the kid that if he fixes that small thing, he won't feel bad. It's bad magic, isn't it? Your child is now working on my tasks, not realizing that I am what is bothering him. This adds to his suffering.

When the mother in this example tried to help her son by taking him into the bathroom and showing him in the mirror that nothing was in his mouth, she unwittingly played into the Dragon's strategy of controlling her son's life. This approach made the son think that if he just looked hard enough into the mirror, he would see the paper. The two of them were then stuck in the bathroom, still upset and unable to enjoy the party. Notice how this plays into the Dragon's plan. The Dragon wants you to focus ever closer on the problem, as the Dragon defines it. If you could just see that paper, the problem would be solved. But this never works, because the paper isn't really there.

When the mother realized that looking in the mirror was getting them nowhere, she tried a new, more successful strategy. Instead of looking into her son's mouth, she said, "This is a Dragon fear. You are way more upset than you would be if this were a simple problem of paper stuck in your mouth. I have heard enough from the Dragon for now. See if you can think of some way to get the Dragon to leave you alone so you can enjoy the party." The son initially resisted this idea, and understandably so. He wanted his fear to be his mother's problem. It was harder having his fear be *his* problem. But he had done a lot of work on other types of anxiety, so he did see her point—that this fear, too, might be anxiety. He tried taking a deep breath and then distracting himself by joining the others in cheering for the child who was hitting the next piñata. Five minutes later his mom saw him running across the lawn, playing soccer with the other kids. His face showed no signs of distress, because the Dragon had given up trying to imprison her son.

## Anxiety Problems Are Neither Rational Nor Fair

Some children are naturally prone to anxiety, while other children are naturally immune to it. Modern research with children shows that these temperamental differences often endure for many years, even for an entire lifetime. Differences are observable in babies under the age of six months. Some newborns startle easily, yet others are almost impervious to changes in their environments, even very loud noises. At the age of two or three, this difference in temperament is seen when children who don't know each other are placed together in unfamiliar settings. Some are fearful and cling to adults, especially to their parents. Other children are immediately happy to find themselves with new playmates.

> All children have different levels of anxiety sensitivity, which is defined as a fearfulness of physical anxiety feelings. Children with high anxiety sensitivity are more likely to have spontaneous panic attacks. (Calamari, et al. *Journal of Behavioral Therapy and Experimental Psychiatry*, vol. 32, no. 3 [September 2001]: 117–36)

A generation or two ago, all childhood behaviors were thought to reflect characteristics of children's interactions with the adults in their lives. Especially important was the "mother–child bond." It was common to explain (or blame) childhood mental disorders on the child's mother. For example, schizophrenia, an especially serious mental disorder, was blamed on disturbed "schizophrenic" mothers. Today few mental health professionals explain childhood mental difficulties this way. In our book, we think of a child's anxiety problems as reflecting how the child's brain works. Most of the differences among children are explained by each child's biology. Parents are clearly important in their children's mental and physical existence, by influencing how their children's biology expresses itself. In other words, adults are not to blame for children's behavioral problems, but they can make problems better or worse by how they handle them.

## Anxiety Is Often a Family Disorder

Anxiety tends to run in families. It is clearly genetic, to a substantial extent. When a child has an anxiety problem, it is common that one of the child's parents also does. Anxiety can often be traced back many generations; it is usually easy to identify family members who were anxious. When there is more than one child in a family, anxiety problems may occur in several of the children, to a greater or a lesser extent. Anxiety also changes over time. In the course of a lifetime, anxiety often shows periods of greater or lesser activity in particular children.

> Another of my best tricks is shifting the anxiety symptoms your child experiences. I don't want you or your child to get too familiar with any of my tricks, because then my tricks wouldn't be a scary surprise. I'm a master of disguise—I have to be, in order to fool your child.

Some people are so troubled by the genetic component of anxiety that they are afraid to have children, lest they pass these anxious tendencies on to another generation. This attitude is too extreme. Remember, anxiety comes in different intensities, from very mild to quite severe. When mild, anxiety could be an advantage to someone leading a successful life, as the person would be likely to think through problems and work hard in school and at his job. The fear of passing along "anxiety genes" to a child is usually a Dragon fear. The Wizard, in contrast, knows that anxious people with some forethought can be successful and happy in their lives.

## Quality People

Here is a surprising fact that we've seen over and over among anxious children and adults. Anxiety tends to go with lots of good characteristics. Anxious people usually want other people to think well of them. They are often obedient and hard-working children.

Anxious children tend to do their homework and their chores around the house. They don't want to be criticized by others, especially by people in authority. Many children refuse to go to school at some point in their lives. Anxious children who refuse to go to

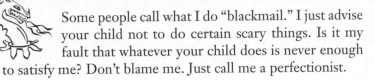

Some people call what I do "blackmail." I just advise your child not to do certain scary things. Is it my fault that whatever your child does is never enough to satisfy me? Don't blame me. Just call me a perfectionist.

school are usually good students when they do attend, whereas truant kids with conduct disorders are usually impulsive and unlikely to do their homework even if they go to school. Kids with conduct disorders typically don't care what adults think about them and often have low grades and lots of behavioral problems in school. All of this is in dramatic contrast to anxious kids. We call anxiety disorders the disorders of quality people because, in general, only the nicest people have them.

## The Bonuses Your Family Can Win by Working on Your Child's Anxiety Problem

This book will guide parents in helping their children overcome the serious negative effects of anxiety in their lives. There are two important bonuses in overcoming anxiety. The first family bonus is that the strategy used here has wide applicability for both the child and the family.

Let's look a bit deeper into the process of recovering from anxiety. The first step is facing and accepting the problem. The problem is real. It needs to be owned, rather than denied or blamed on others. The second step is to get help from everyone who can help. This includes help from this book, as well as from family members. The third step is to put into practice the experts' suggestions and do the hard work necessary to truly solve the problem. The fourth step is to commit the family to a lifelong process of working to manage the problem. Since the anxiety problem is likely to be lifelong, so must the work to stay well be lifelong. This four-step recovery program will prove useful in dealing not only with anxiety, but with medical illnesses; relationship, school, and employment problems; and lots of other serious issues that will arise for your family.

## A Bonus-Bonus

Beyond this bonus is a second benefit from following this book's advice. Many anxious children have parents with significant anxiety problems. Some of these parents have not adequately dealt with their own anxiety. The family team strategy in this book works for the whole family, not just for the anxious child. Parents who are devoted to helping their children will find that they can at long last deal successfully with their own anxiety problems. If you, as a parent, do not have anxiety, then you can use this book's problem-solving strategy on your other problems. All families have real and serious problems for which this four-step strategy will be effective.

That Dragon can be a big problem for your child. If she does the Dragon's bidding, she will suffer terribly and her life will be crippled. I have lots of magic to help you get the Dragon out of your child's life. Powerful magic takes hard work over a long period of time. My magic is not easy, but it is strong.

## Getting Help from Professionals and Antianxiety Medications

Another dimension in the process of getting well needs to be dealt with at the outset. When and how should you use professional mental health providers, medications, or both to deal with your child's anxiety problems? There are no hard-and-fast rules, but we have found two principles useful in answering this question. The first is that if the anxiety problem is especially severe—that is, if it has a major impact on your child's activities and causes serious distress for your child and your family—then it's a good idea to get help from a mental health professional right away. Later, we will describe how to do this most effectively, to ensure a positive outcome.

The second principle is to start with what the family can do on its own, by using the techniques that you'll learn here. Whatever you decide about using professional mental health treatment, the techniques in this book will surely prove useful. We, the authors, are active in our own mental health practices. We use medications with many of our child patients. We are in favor of using both professional mental health treatment and medication. Yet therapy and medications are seldom enough to produce a full, robust recovery from anxiety problems. Getting well usually requires family members working together, using the techniques we describe in this book. Anxiety problems tend to be lifelong, while professional therapy is almost always relatively brief or perhaps intermittent over the years. Your family will be on its own a good deal of the time when coping with anxiety.

I can be harsh, but when tamed I actually become useful. Are you willing to work hard and long enough with your child? Can you transform me from a bad guy into a not-so-bad guy and maybe even into a good guy?

The use of antianxiety medications, though possibly an important part of your child's life, is often episodic as well. This means that a lot of time will be spent dealing with anxiety without the help of medications. That is one more good reason to take advantage of the techniques you'll find in this book.

Many people who worry too much—people with anxiety problems—are reluctant to use formal mental health treatment and modern antianxiety medications. That is hardly surprising, because results from these methods are uncertain and controversy and disagreement abound in regard to their effectiveness. We are not afraid of using mental health treatment or medications with children. We encourage you not to be afraid of them, either. We often remind our patients that treatment and medications are not like brain surgery. If you don't like the results, you can always stop the treatment or the medication and go back to the way you were. The only acceptable standard that makes sense in judging the efficacy of treatment or medication is whether they make your child's and your family's lives better.

## Using the Family Team

In this book we write about the "family team." We, the three authors of this book, are a family, working together in our mental health practices to solve anxiety problems. With most of our adult patients and all of our child patients, we find that working with entire families is essential for everyone to get the most out of treatment. The number one goal of a family team is to help the children grow up, leave the parents' home, and form their own careers and families. Anxiety can thwart that process and limit children's achievements. Families need to confront a child's anxiety and do whatever it takes to solve the anxiety problem.

## A "Cure" from Anxiety

Now you know that anxiety runs in families and that over time it tends to wax and wane in a child's life, but anxiety is unlikely to ever go away entirely (although sometimes this does happen). No treatment will take away anxious feelings entirely forever, although many treatments do a lot of good in lowering the intensity of anxiety and eliminating the disability often caused by anxiety. Everyone with an anxiety problem, including children, needs to be prepared for anxiety to return at any time. This is the way the Dragon works. It will hide for a long time, hoping you'll forget the techniques you used to solve your problem. Once you forget these techniques, the Dragon will use its own cunning tricks, like its incredible ability to disguise itself as something it is not. Maybe you will see the Dragon as a dreaded physical illness that shocks you back into prison with a sneak attack.

Given those facts, which can sound darn gloomy, how are we so bold as to offer a "cure"? A cure means knowing what is wrong and what to do about any problem. When a person understands the nature of the anxiety from which she suffers and also knows what to do about it, the process of cure is well underway. When that person does what she knows will work—even though it takes a lot of effort over a long period of time—then she not only lessens the pain of the anxiety problem, but she totally overcomes all of the disability resulting from it. As a bonus, the person also experiences a huge boost in self-esteem, which comes from doing a difficult job well. Curing oneself is like winning an Olympic gold medal. It takes years of hard work and a lot of understanding. The entire family can happily share that wonderful feeling of accomplishment. This is a gold medal for your family team.

### Action Steps

- Keep an eye on how scared the Dragon is making YOU. If you're scared, it will be hard to help your child.
- Use the calm, confident voice of the Wizard to help your child learn to think about solving his Dragon problem.

CHAPTER 4

# Evaluating Your Child's Need for Medication and Therapy

Anxiety is made up of feelings, thoughts, and behaviors. You and your child will want to work on all three of these. We are giving you the tools you need to reduce or eliminate your child's anxiety. Many people will need no more than their new knowledge and the tools they'll find in this book to conquer their anxiety problems.

It is also true, however, that many parents work diligently with these tools, yet nevertheless continue to struggle because their children are so seriously handicapped by anxiety. Some children are unable to even begin the work recommended in this book because they are so overwhelmed by anxiety. We recognize that many parents have found this book after being in therapy with their children and after using medications to reduce the children's anxiety. Thus, they are already familiar with these treatments. Yet even parents whose children do not need medications or therapy will find it useful to understand what these interventions offer. We want our readers to understand how antianxiety medications work, what they do, and what they don't do. We also want everyone to realize what modern therapy can and cannot do. Finally, we offer practical suggestions on finding, using, and evaluating medications and therapy for your anxious child.

Parents have a hard job in helping a child overcome anxiety problems. If you feel overwhelmed by the challenge, find a therapist who can help you do this work. You may want to see a therapist together with your child, or you alone could get help in guiding your child's progress. A therapist or a psychiatrist can also evaluate your child if you're unsure whether you are dealing with an anxiety problem.

## The History of Antianxiety Medications

For more than a hundred years, doctors have known that sedating medicines reduce anxiety. Beginning in the second decade of the twentieth century, doctors frequently prescribed one of a family of new synthetic sedatives called barbiturates. These were all chemical modifications of barbituric acid. The problem with these medications, which worked similarly to alcohol, was that they produced sedation and even poor coordination at doses that significantly reduced anxiety. In addition, they were potentially fatal when taken in overdoses, and they were abused by alcoholics and drug addicts.

Then in 1961 the first of an entirely new kind of antianxiety medication was introduced, Librium (chlordiazepoxide). Two years later Valium (diazepam) was marketed in the United States as the first widely used antianxiety medication since barbiturates came on the scene half a century earlier. These new medications, called benzodiazepines, were a huge improvement over the earlier ones used to quiet the nervous system. They reduced anxiety at doses that didn't cause sedation or disturb motor coordination. They were not fatal in overdose situations.

As good as these medications were, however, they weren't perfect. The most serious problem was that doctors didn't recognize or understand anxiety disorders, as we do now, so these medications were often prescribed without clear indications for their use, leading to widespread overuse by people who didn't have serious anxiety problems. Alcoholics and drug addicts also abused the benzodiazepines. This created another set of difficulties. Nevertheless, the benzodiazepines were frequently used and were generally very helpful to many anxious patients.

Before the late 1950s, the only treatments available for depression were electroshock and other risky methods such as insulin coma therapy. Then researchers discovered a medication that successfully treated depression: imipramine. Called Tofranil, it revolutionized thinking in the field. In 1959 a pioneer in biological psychiatry, Dr. Donald Klein, observed that imipramine not only treated depression but blocked panic attacks as well. He also made the remarkable discovery that people with agoraphobia often suffered from fear of panic attacks. This led to his understanding that imipramine could treat agoraphobia, even in the absence of depression. Not many years later, Dr. Klein discovered that school phobia, based on fear of separation from a parent, was analogous to agoraphobia in adults and that it, too, could be successfully treated with imipramine.

There were significant problems with imipramine, helpful as it was for the anxiety disorders. Imipramine was hard for patients to tolerate because of its bothersome side effects, such as sedation, dry mouth, constipation, urinary retention, and weight gain. It produced cardiac problems, especially in children and the elderly, some of which were fatal. In addition, imipramine and other tricyclic antidepressants (TCAs) were sometimes fatal in overdose situations.

The introduction of a new generation of antidepressants in the late 1980s—of which Prozac, Zoloft, and Paxil were the most prominent examples—revolutionized not only the treatment of depression but also that of anxiety disorders. Unlike the TCAs, the new antidepressants, callled SSRIs as a class, were easier for patients to use, had fewer annoying side effects, and were not fatal in overdose situations. Unlike the benzodiazepines, they had no abuse potential for drug addicts and alcoholics. Though initially introduced for adults, these classes of antianxiety medications, the benzodiazepines and the antidepressants, were soon discovered to be equally safe and effective for children. There are two primary reasons to use medications in the treatment of crippling anxiety. The first and most basic is to quiet the overactive, sensitized nervous system and to block the panic attacks that are at the heart of many anxiety disorders. The second reason is to give anxiety sufferers some measure of control over their symptoms. Just knowing that the medications work can be a tremendous boost to self-confidence and a basis for hope, which might motivate people to work hard to overcome their anxiety problems.

A study of children/adolescents with PTSD, compared to adults with PTSD, found that the children/adolescents and the adults all improved significantly over the course of the eight-week-long study when treated with selective serotonin reuptake inhibitors (SSRIs). The findings are so clear, it is likely that PTSD is caused by a brain chemistry imbalance that the SSRI corrects. (Seedat, et al. *Journal of Child and Adolescent Psychopharmacology*, vol. 12, no. 1 [Spring 2002]: 37–46)

## Current Medicines

Today the antidepressants and the benzodiazepines are still the two classes of medicines that are widely used to treat clinically significant anxiety in children and adults. They are used separately or together, or are combined with other medications. Antipsychotics, antiseizure medicines, and mood stabilizers, among others, are sometimes added to boost the effectiveness of the medicines used to treat anxious children. This does not necessarily mean that a child has an additional mental health diagnosis. These supplemental medicines are generally used only after the antidepressants and the benzodiazepines have been found to not work effectively on their own. Children who are already taking medicines to treat ADHD may benefit from also using either or both of these classes of medicines, usually without problems. Decisions about medication must be made with a doctor who knows your child well and who is familiar with these medicines.

The antidepressants were initially introduced, as their name indicates, to treat depression. Most have been found to be effective in treating anxiety disorders. They are a good first choice for anxious children, especially when depression occurs along with the anxiety and the anxiety is an everyday problem. The antidepressants are usually taken once a day for six months or longer, and they generally take several weeks of regular use to become effective.

The benzodiazepines, in contrast, work within a half hour of their being taken. Their antianxiety benefits last about four to eight hours. An extended-release form of Xanax, called Xanax XR, has recently been introduced. It has less of a sedative effect and needs to be taken only once a day compared to three or four times per day for immediate-release Xanax. Benzodiazepines can be taken only as needed or several times a day, every day.

In both the benzodiazepines and the antidepressants, the side effects are usually medically trivial and disappear after a few days or weeks of use. Extensive studies of the use of antidepressants and the benzodiazepines by children have begun only within the past few years, but these medicines have been carefully studied in adults for decades. They have been shown to be generally safe even in long-term use. There is sound reason to expect that the same safety profile will be found for children. Because these medicines are widely used, they are the subjects of active research. If problems were to be found in children using them, they would certainly be well publicized. These prescription medicines must be prescribed by a physician, who will be actively involved in educating you about the safety profile of each medicine.

We prescribe the antidepressants and the benzodiazepines for many of the anxious children we treat. We seldom see significant side effects and are comfortable with both short-term and long-term uses of these medicines. Extended-release formulations of many of the antidepressants have recently become available. There are even newer antianxiety medicines being developed that have entirely different mechanisms of action. Because we conduct clinical trials of new medications, we are confident that the extensive anxiety disorder research in basic science and clinical practice will lead to even better antianxiety medicines for children in the future.

## The History of Therapy as a Treatment of Anxiety

The therapy scene for anxiety disorders had a similar evolution over this same period of time. Throughout most of the twentieth century, the standard method of treating anxiety disorders was psychoanalytic psychotherapy, which focused on working through unconscious conflicts that involved repressed angry and sexual feelings. This approach didn't work well with most anxious patients, although some benefited from it. In the late 1970s a new form of therapy was pioneered in academic psychology: cognitive behavioral treatment (CBT). Unlike traditional psychotherapy, CBT focused on teaching patients techniques for changing their thoughts and behaviors, with the assumption that when these changed, the feelings would, too.

Unrelated to this academic track, a group of clinical practitioners developed a new form of therapy, which was sometimes called contextual therapy or supported exposure therapy. This treatment, often done in groups with anxiety patients and their families, used techniques to change both thoughts and behaviors, with the underlying message being that patients need not fear their uncomfortable feelings and not avoid whatever their anxious feelings told them to avoid. In the 1990s this new form of mental health treatment became widespread in the United States. The purpose of modern therapy for anxiety disorders is to arm the patient with effective techniques to handle anxiety as it appears. These techniques employ both cognitive and behavioral strategies, as well as many related activities to bolster self-confidence and reduce tension, such as regular aerobic exercise. We incorporated these techniques in this book, which makes it a useful supplement to all forms of therapy for anxiety disorders.

Interestingly, after the new medications and forms of treatment were widely and effectively put to use, "insight-oriented psychotherapy" or "dynamic psychotherapy" (the direct descendant of the earlier psychoanalytic psychotherapy) could play a new role in anxious people's lives.

## The Meaning of Therapy and Medication

Many parents have very strong feelings about considering medication or therapy for their child. These may stem from various concerns—for example, a reluctance to label the child with a psychiatric diagnosis, a fear of the long-term effects of medication, or a general disbelief in the benefits of therapy. If you feel uncomfortable with these topics, you might want to ask yourself what aspect of this process of getting help for your child upsets you. On the other hand, some parents are very hopeful that medications or therapy will solve the problem right away, and they're eager to get started. As with many situations, the reality is somewhere in-between. Taking medication or going to therapy will neither make a child sick nor change the reality of his suffering. These methods are not magic bullets, either. Rarely is education or therapy a cure-all, but each strategy could solve a piece of the puzzle.

> Medication, psychiatrists, therapy . . . so many more things I can scare your child with! Think of all the "What if" anxieties I can grow from those seeds in your anxious child's mind. Of course, if you and your child actually know something about these topics, I have a harder time scaring either of you.

The question is, "Does your child need professional help?" A psychiatrist, a psychologist, or a social worker could help in several ways. The first important step in evaluating the need for medication or therapy is to identify the diagnosis. This may be fairly straightforward. You may already have a pretty good idea what type of anxiety your child has, or it may be a diagnostic challenge to sort out the different issues. An anxiety disorder may be a single diagnosis, or there may be more than one problem. For example, depression or attention deficit hyperactivity disorder (ADHD) may be confounding the problem. It may not be possible for you to figure this out, and you shouldn't have to do it alone.

When a professional sees your child for the first time, that individual will help clarify your child's diagnosis. The next step is to identify the goals of the treatment. Is the main goal immediate symptom relief? Or is it ongoing treatment, with slow, steady improvement over weeks and months? If the goal is immediate relief, the options are somewhat different from those for ongoing treatment. This chapter is divided into these two categories, which in turn are divided into medication and therapy sections. Some kids will benefit from both immediate and long-term treatment, while others need only one or the other.

> Medications can turn down the brain's danger alarm. That can make it a lot easier for your child to use the magic from this book. It's hard for your child to face his fears when he is overwhelmed by intense, biologically caused panic. (U.S. Department of Health and Human Services. *Mental Health: A Report of the Surgeon General*, 1999)

## Immediate Symptom Relief

### Medication

Parents are generally less worried about this topic, because they are so eager to do whatever it takes to help their child who is suffering from high levels of anxiety. The need for immediate symptom relief is so clear. This visit to a psychiatrist or a pediatrician often comes up in a crisis situation. The child is suffering and the parents are upset. They feel that nothing they do is helping. For example, Lucy was starting first grade. She had been nervous about starting school all summer, but her mom thought that it was a normal reaction for such a big step. As the first day of school approached, Lucy became more and more upset. Each night she asked many questions about school but didn't seem to be reassured by her mom's answers.

Two nights before school started, Lucy couldn't sleep. She clung to her mom and cried all night long. Her mother continued trying to reassure Lucy, but with no success. The next morning they were both exhausted. Lucy said she was *not* going to go to school the following day. Lucy's mom felt terrible about her inability to solve this problem. She was worried that she would have to make a terrible choice: either force Lucy, kicking and screaming, to go to school, or keep her home and hope that the next day would be better. She called the pediatrician, who prescribed an antianxiety medication. Lucy took the medication that night and slept well for the first time in three nights. The next morning she was a little apprehensive but not overwhelmed. She took the medication again with breakfast and left for school feeling excited but not anxious. She continued the medication during the first week of school. After that, she didn't need it anymore. She had no further trouble going to school.

The medication the pediatrician prescribed for Lucy was in the group called benzodiazepines. These include Valium (diazepam), Klonopin (clonazepam), Ativan (lorazepam), and Xanax (alprazolam). People often think of these as sedatives. They do have a sedative effect at higher doses, but at lower doses there is a direct antianxiety effect without sedation for most people. These medications have been well studied and are safe and effective in treating anxiety of any cause. They reduce anxiety. It doesn't matter if the person has an anxiety disorder (a diagnosable illness) or not. They

Side effects of antianxiety medications are another great opportunity for me to make you and your child worry. Side effects are a terrific topic for anxiety because until your child actually takes a medication, even your doctor doesn't know which particular side effect may occur in your child. Of course, most kids take medications for anxiety these days with no side effects at all, and any problems that do occur are not dangerous—but I never mention that.

also work quickly, often within fifteen to twenty minutes. This is why it was such a good choice for Lucy. The day before school starts is not the time to do an extensive diagnostic evaluation for an anxiety disorder. The most important thing for her doctor to do was help Lucy calm down so that she wouldn't miss school. Medication for a short period was all that she needed. In some cases, though, use of a benzodiazepine may be a first step, and the child might need further support to continue in school.

There are two drawbacks to these benzodiazepine medications, neither of which is usually a problem for anxious disorders. The main problem is that people with a drug addiction or alcoholism can abuse these medications. At higher doses they can have an intoxicating effect. People who abuse benzodiazepines take higher and higher doses to get a euphoric feeling, which is essentially like being drunk. This is not a problem for most people with anxiety, who don't want a euphoric feeling. For most anxious people, feeling drunk is terribly unpleasant. They just want to feel "normal" and want to get on with their lives. The parents can easily monitor their child's use of these medications. The second problem is the potential for physical dependence. This means that if people take a sufficient dose of the medication every day for many weeks, they might have physical withdrawal symptoms if the medication is stopped abruptly. This is generally not a problem for children being treated for anxiety, for three reasons. First, the dose is generally low enough for them to stop without a problem, even after prolonged everyday use. Second, the medications are generally taken only for a short time. Third, even if the medication is taken consistently, when it's time to stop, you simply taper the dose down gradually over a couple of weeks to avoid withdrawal symptoms. The main reason we even mention these issues is that you may already have heard something about them. For example, Lucy was fortunate that her pediatrician was experienced in the use of these medications; he explained the issues of abuse and dependence to Lucy's father, who had heard that these medications were dangerous. Once Lucy's father understood these facts he was no longer afraid to let Lucy use a benzodiazepine.

### Medicines Used to Treat Anxiety in Children

| Type of Medicine | Advantages | Disadvantages |
| --- | --- | --- |
| Antidepressants | Taken twice a day<br>Treat both anxiety and depression | May take weeks of daily use to work<br>Usually taken for months or years |
| Benzodiazepines | Act immediately<br>Can be used only when needed | Abused by people addicted to alcohol and other drugs<br>Should be discontinued gradually after daily use |

Many children with anxiety problems do well without using any antianxiety medicines. When anxiety is severe and persistent despite nonmedication efforts to overcome it, using one of the antidepressants or a benzodiazepine to reduce the anxiety becomes an option to consider. Medicines often permit a severely anxious child to benefit from other forms of treatment, including the techniques in this book. Talking with a therapist about using medicines can be enormously helpful for both anxious children and their parents. Selecting specific medicines and managing their use requires working with a medical doctor, often a pediatrician, a child psychiatrist, or another physician familiar with the treatment of anxiety problems in children. If the first medicine your child tries does not produce the desired results, it is comforting to recognize that there are now more than a dozen medicines available to use to safely and effectively reduce anxiety in children.

## Therapy

Often our first contact with children and their families comes at a time of crisis, when they are looking for immediate relief. Most families leave that first session feeling better, even though we have only just met them. Two important things can be communicated in only a short time: that it's possible to become educated about anxiety and that you can use special tools to diminish anxiety. We teach you these skills in this book. You don't need to see a professional to learn these techniques. However, it can be helpful to have another player on your team, to help tailor a plan specifically for your child. It's especially important to get a professional diagnosis if your child is missing school or falling rapidly behind in one or more areas because of anxiety. It isn't unusual for a family to come into our office only a few times to get started. Seeing a therapist need not be a long-term commitment.

## Ongoing Treatment

In this section, we don't recommend that therapy be for any specific length of time or imply a commitment to long-term treatment. We are merely discussing nonimmediate or noncrisis treatment. Many options are available, including self-help (like this book), medication, and therapy. Making a decision to start a child on medication or therapy can be hard. Remember, these are not permanent decisions. They are simply options for your family to consider. Trying medication is not a commitment to lifelong treatment or a sign of serious mental illness.

### Medication

Anxiety disorders are serious problems. The cost of not treating an anxiety disorder can be very high. Anxious children tend to develop low self-esteem and become socially isolated. They even have more physical problems, like headaches and stomach aches. Many parents are focused on the risks of using medications, but we think it's also important to look at the risk of *not* using medications. Katie's story is a good example. Imagine what might have happened had she not received help so quickly.

Fourteen-year-old Katie had always been a worrier. At times, this was a problem. She saw a therapist for a short period last year. That was helpful, because she learned some useful strategies to cope with her periods of anxiety. About four months ago Katie had her first panic attack. She was going to a friend's house to study for a test, when the Dragon hit her. She had never felt so afraid. She had a racing heart, was trembling and dizzy, and thought she might die. Her mother was so frightened by Katie's symptoms that she brought her daughter to the emergency room. There Katie had a physical exam, an electrocardiogram, and laboratory tests. Everything was fine. The doctor told her that it was probably a panic attack. He sent Katie home with a small number of Xanax tablets and instructions to call her pediatrician if the symptoms recurred. Katie was fine for about a week, and then it happened again. She was home at the time, so she took one of the Xanax tablets. She soon felt better but then began to worry that she would have more panic attacks. She canceled her weekend plans, telling her mother that she wished she didn't have to go to school the following week. Her mother took Katie back to see the therapist. This helped, but she continued to have panic attacks. The therapist recommended a psychiatrist to prescribe medications. Katie was very upset by this. "She thinks I'm crazy!" "No," said her mother, "she thinks you are suffering."

### The Benzodiazepines

| Generic Names | Trade Names |
| --- | --- |
| alprazolam | Xanax |
| clonazepam | Klonopin |
| diazepam | Valium |
| extended-release alprazolam | Xanax XR |
| lorazepam | Ativan |

The psychiatrist diagnosed her with panic disorder and prescribed an antidepressant medication called Zoloft. He explained that it might take three to six weeks before the medication really started working. Katie noticed a change for the better in about two weeks. After a month of taking Zoloft, she was convinced. Not only did she have fewer panic attacks, but she worried much less than before. She didn't feel drugged and told her doctor, "I feel like my old self, but even better because I'm not worried all the time." Zoloft is just one in a group of medications commonly used to treat anxiety disorders. These medications were first used as antidepressants, but they all have independent antianxiety properties.

*The Antidepressants*

| Generic Names | Trade Names |
|---|---|
| buspirone | Buspar |
| clomipramine | Anafranil |
| citalopram | Celexa |
| escitalopram | Lexapro |
| fluoxetine | Prozac |
| fluvoxamine | Luvox |
| imipramine | Tofranil |
| mirtazapine | Remeron |
| nefazodone | Serzone |
| nortriptyline | Pamelor |
| paroxetine | Paxil |
| sertraline | Zoloft |
| venlafaxine | Effexor |

The main class of antidepressant medications for the treatment of anxiety is the selective serotonin reuptake inhibitors (SSRIs). These medications make more serotonin available for the neurons in the brain to keep the amount of serotonin at a normal level. They do not have antianxiety effects for people who don't have an anxiety disorder, nor do they have abuse or dependence potential. The medications in this group are Prozac (fluoxetine), Paxil (paroxetine), Zoloft (sertraline), Celexa (citalopram), Luvox (fluvoxamine), and Lexapro (escitalopram). Several other antidepressant medications have slightly different mechanisms of action but are still commonly used for the treatment of anxiety; these include Effexor (venlafaxine), Remeron (mirtazapine), Pamelor (nortriptyline), and Serzone (nefazedone). The antidepressants have become the most common first choice for treatment of anxiety because they are effective, safe, and easy to use and have few side effects.

Research shows that, in general, the SSRIs and similar new anti-depressant medications are equally effective in treating children's anxiety. However, an individual may find one of these medications superior to another. The best thing about these medicines is that once they take effect, they work twenty-four hours a day. There is no need to guess whether or when you'll have an anxious experience. The worst thing about these medications is that they take several weeks to start making a difference.

Another thing I never tell anxious people is that any medication side effects are easily handled by staying at the same dose for a few more days and waiting for your child's body to get used to the medicine. If that doesn't work, your doctor may suggest lowering the dose or even stopping the medication and trying another one. The side effects don't last after the medication is stopped. Thinking about possible side effects provides many great "What ifs" that I can scare you and your child with! I'm nasty—but you knew that already.

The benzodiazepines can be used for ongoing treatment as well. They are particularly helpful for episodic, anticipated anxiety because they work quickly, unlike the SSRIs. For example, Rachel was not afraid of anything, except flying. As long as no air travel was in her future, she was fine. However, she was really terrified of flying. She wanted to use the self-help model for treatment and had just gotten started with a plan of gradually desensitizing herself to airports. Then she was offered a chance to go to Europe for the summer with a school friend. She was very eager to go, but how could she fly across the ocean? This trip included no less than four flights! She continued her practice but also got a prescription for

Klonopin. She had ten pills for her monthlong trip. She decided to try to fly without taking the medications but wanted to bring the pills along as a backup plan. She took one pill before her first flight. Then she realized that she was having such a great time, she didn't need any pills for the rest of the trip. "But I knew I could take it if I wanted to, and that made a big difference." Rachel returned to her doctor two years later. She had done a lot of traveling and had used only a few of those ten original pills. She was now about to start college in a distant state. She would be flying a lot, so she decided to get some new pills, "just in case."

All of the medications in this chapter are used for both adults and children. There is good research supporting their use in treating childhood anxiety. However, most medications have not been specifically approved by the FDA for pediatric use. This is disturbing to many parents. Unfortunately, it's expensive and time-consuming for pharmaceutical companies to conduct pediatric clinical trials. A significant number of medications are currently being studied for children and more will follow, as there is a lot of interest in children's anxiety. The available research reassures us that these medications are generally safe and effective for children.

## Therapy

The main form of therapy for anxiety problems is cognitive-behavioral therapy, or CBT, whether for short- or long-term treatment. If your child has just a few sessions of therapy during an anxiety crisis, these would focus primarily on education and on reframing the problem. Having six or more sessions with a therapist could allow much more work to be done. A therapist will typically help a child with the cognitive part of this approach by teaching him how to change his thinking about his disorder and his symptoms. For example, the mantra "My anxiety is distressing but not dangerous" expresses the central idea that the anxiety Dragon's only weapon is discomfort. The way the Dragon gets its power is by implying that its powers extend well beyond mere discomfort. The false alarm of anxiety leads, naturally enough, to the conviction that the panic and anxiety will surely cause grave consequences, such as heart attacks, strokes, seizures, madness, and other stress-related disorders—even sudden death. To the extent that the anxiety sufferer can believe, really believe, that all the anxiety can do is make him temporarily uncomfortable, the key element of the Dragon's power is neutralized. The way the Dragon does its work is by inducing intense "What if" fears. Those fears further sensitize the anxious mind and greatly heighten and prolong the suffering from anxiety. Dozens of other cognitive techniques in this book are widely used. For example, noting your anxiety level from 1 to 10 objectifies the anxiety and helps you become a student of the disorder. This shifts the experience from one of victimization to one of thoughtful observation. Remember, the panic always goes down if the sufferer doesn't run but just holds her ground.

In a longer-term relationship with a therapist, there is also time to work on the behavioral aspects of the problem. Anxiety induces avoidance of the source of the fear. This avoidance produces a short-term drop in panic and anxiety. The anxious person learns that when he runs from the Dragon, the symptoms lessen. What is not learned is that the Dragon is a blackmailer and it merely appears more often when the anxiety sufferer avoids things that are important in his life. The second lesson to learn is that avoidance is not necessary for the anxiety and panic to fade. All that you need is time. Panic cannot be sustained; the alarm fades eventually, even without avoiding the scary situation. So the behavioral component of this therapy is to move toward your fears and not away from them. That movement can be fast or slow. It can be alone or with someone else. For most anxious children, this process of confronting fears is best done slowly and in the presence of a sympathetic and supportive adult. Most often, this would be the child's parent.

In addition to trying CBT, it's often helpful for anxious children and their parents to work with a professional therapist. Partly, this is because the therapist has good ideas and is a trusted guide to rely upon. And, partly, it's helpful because therapy provides a place for the child and the parent to talk about other important things that don't exclusively relate to anxiety.

# Psychologists, Psychiatrists, and Social Workers

Usually, anxiety is a long-term problem, although sometimes it goes away. When it does go away, it often returns, even years later—but not always. To the extent that anxiety persists or else leaves and returns, the child has multiple opportunities to cope with it over a long period of time. This gives the child and her parents time to try many ways of dealing with the problem. If the anxiety is severe, if it persists, or if it doesn't quickly fade when you use the techniques recommended here, by all means do seek out a therapist, a physician, or both, who can prescribe antianxiety medications. Even if you don't stick with either therapy or medication for a long period of time, you owe it to yourself and your child to try these approaches. They are often tremendously helpful, and you won't know how helpful until you try them.

Today most therapists are not physicians; they are usually either psychologists (often Ph.D.'s) or social workers (M.S.W.'s). These people are likely to work in fifty-minute hours, seeing a child and his parents once a week—sometimes more often and sometimes less often—for months or even years. In the later stages of therapy, visits may be infrequent—say, once a month or even once in three months. Most therapists are connected with physicians who prescribe medications for children with anxiety problems. So it usually makes sense to find a therapist first and then have the therapist refer you to a doctor who prescribes medications. Often this is a child psychiatrist, but it can be a pediatrician who is comfortable dealing with anxiety problems.

Usually, your child will see the prescribing doctor much less often than the therapist. At first, there may be a fifty-minute interview, to establish the diagnosis and develop the initial treatment plan. Because anxiety is often a family disease, the doctor is likely to ask if other family members have an anxiety problem and whether any medications or other treatments have been helpful. This can be a guide to what will work with your child because people in the same family often react similarly to various medications. In the past, psychiatrists both prescribed medications and offered therapy; some still do and they are not always gray-haired. This can be a very effective strategy, although it has become less common.

You will need to keep careful track of the medications your child tries. Set up a chart in your child's Journal to record the doctor's name, medication names, dates, doses, side effects, and whether the medication was helpful. This will save you an enormous amount of trouble in the future if you end up seeing different doctors and therapists. You may think that you'll never forget the name of the wonderful medication that saved your child during an anxiety crisis, but a few years from now, if your child is in another crisis, it will be much better to have everything clearly recorded in your child's Journal.

Your child's pediatrician can refer you to a therapist and or a child psychiatrist. You can also contact the Anxiety Disorders Association of America for information about therapists in your area. Your child's school counselors and nursing staff may have recommendations, too. When you do make an appointment, give the person a chance to help. Therapists and doctors work differently, and no one approach works best for all anxious children. If the therapist or doctor you've chosen doesn't help within a few visits, you might think about trying someone else. We have found that improvements come early, at least to a limited degree. Over time, the standard to apply to therapy and medication is that they should help your child cope more successfully with anxiety. If they don't, look around for a better fit for your particular needs.

When we talk about therapy in this book, we generally mean cognitive behavioral therapy. Other types of therapy are available but systematic studies have shown not only efficacy but sustained response with CBT. A medication lasts only as long as it is taken, but benefits from CBT can endure long after therapy has ended.

### Action Steps

- If you are in doubt about your child's need for medication or therapy, go to a therapist yourself to ask more questions and to describe your child's anxiety problem. Let that person, who has experience with anxious kids and worried parents, help you decide on the next best step.

- Meeting with a therapist or psychiatrist doesn't worsen your child's anxiety problem. You are merely reaching out to get additional help to better cope with your child's suffering.

## PART TWO

# *Five Stories for Kids, Five Steps for Parents*

CHAPTER 5

# Step 1

*Ben's Story—Understanding
Your Child's Dragon*

Ben was twelve when we met him. He had wavy brown hair and chocolate brown eyes that often looked worried. His dad said that Ben thought about things too much. His mom wondered why Ben was afraid of school on Monday morning, even though he liked his teacher and all of his homework was finished and ready to be turned in.

Ben was a really good boy and a very good student. He could never explain to adults why lots of things were scary to him, because he knew that these things didn't scare other people. Even his ten-year-old sister went to movies that Ben was too scared to see. It was embarrassing. Ben felt like he was the only kid in the world who worried like this. Thinking about how much he worried made Ben even more scared. He could see no way out of his fears. He tried to stay home from school as much as possible, but then his teachers called a special meeting with his parents. They warned his family that Ben would be held back a year if he missed any more school without a doctor's note.

Ben's parents took him to see a psychiatrist, a doctor who helps kids with difficult feelings like intense fear and sadness. The psychiatrist talked to Ben for a while and told him to imagine that he had a big, mean Dragon in his head. Every time Ben tried to do something the Dragon didn't want him to do, the Dragon would growl and breathe fire. The Dragon's fire, naturally, scared Ben all the more. Ben would do almost anything to avoid making the Dragon mad. The doctor explained that the imaginary Dragon wanted Ben to be scared, because the Dragon ate Ben's fear. Actually, Ben's fear was the only food that the Dragon could eat. The more Ben feared the Dragon, the bigger and scarier it grew. The doctor mentioned something that Ben had already noticed—the Dragon couldn't really hurt him. Oh, sure, the Dragon could make him feel really, really scared. The Dragon made him tremble and feel sick to his stomach, but that was it. The Dragon couldn't keep Ben from doing things. It could never make Ben feel any worse than he had already felt. Ben could walk and talk, play and go to school, even if the Dragon was breathing fire. When the Dragon was mad, it made these things hard for Ben to do. But, with extra effort, Ben could still do whatever he wanted, even when the Dragon was very mad.

The doctor said that the Dragon wanted Ben to put himself into the Dragon's prison—a place where Ben was allowed to do only a few things and was forbidden to do many others. To keep Ben in prison, the Dragon got mad, to make Ben feel bad. The Dragon didn't want Ben to escape by going to school, staying at a friend's house, or going on a school field trip. Even when Ben did everything the Dragon told him to do, that nasty Dragon wouldn't leave Ben alone. The more Ben feared the Dragon and gave in to it, the more of Ben's life the Dragon wanted. The Dragon didn't play fair.

The psychiatrist said that there was good news about the Dragon, too. The Dragon wasn't really able to do what it threatened to do. The Dragon could make Ben feel scared but couldn't hurt him. Also, the more that Ben did, even though he was scared, the smaller the Dragon would get because then Ben wasn't feeding the hungry Dragon. If Ben stopped feeding the Dragon, it would wither away out of neglect.

The doctor said he would help Ben use the Wizard in his head, the Wizard who could teach Ben techniques to tame the Dragon.

The Dragon wanted to be in charge of Ben, but the Wizard could teach Ben so many tricks that the Dragon could never be in charge. Ben would be in charge, and the good Wizard would help him.

Ben felt better as he left the doctor that day. He thought about how the Dragon tried to keep him from going to school, even though he really liked school. His parents didn't understand why he was afraid because they didn't know about his Dragon. They couldn't see or hear it, as Ben could. It made sense to Ben that the fear that he was scared of was all in his own mind. This explained why other people weren't afraid. After all, none of his friends were scared to go to school. Some days they liked school and some days they didn't, but they were never scared to go to school. Ben had that Dragon in his head, but they didn't, so they weren't afraid of the things that scared Ben.

The next day Ben again felt scared when he got ready for school. He took a big drink of orange juice, as he thought about what the doctor had said about the Dragon. Then he tried a Wizard trick. He said to himself, "Dragon, this is my day to go to school. I like school, and I want to stay with my grade, so I'm going, no matter what you do to me." Ben immediately felt better! The Dragon got smaller and quieter. Ben said good-bye to his mother and ran to the bus stop, without feeling sick to his stomach for the first time in months. It felt great to climb on the school bus and sit next to his friend Anton without being scared. Ben felt like he had escaped from the Dragon's prison.

While he was at school, Ben decided that the fierce Dragon needed a name to make it seem less scary. Since his best friend was named Anton, Ben named his Dragon Antwerp. This, he felt, showed the Dragon that they could work at being friends, but that Ben wouldn't be afraid of the Dragon anymore. He wasn't afraid of his friends.

Ben still had to do more work to get over his Dragon attacks, but he was on his way to feeling a lot better once he learned that Antwerp couldn't hurt him, and that Antwerp would shrink if it couldn't eat his fear. Ben had already taken control. The Dragon no longer ran Ben's life; Ben did.

## Step 1: Study Your Child's Dragon

We want you to become a student of your child's fear. Many parents come into our office believing that they understand their kid's fears, but what they really see is the child's troublesome outward behavior, not the inner process that drives it. Understanding why your child acts this way is important and takes less effort than you may imagine. It requires changing your focus, and your child's focus, from the first moment that anxiety becomes unmanageable. To do this, you must help your child understand how to rate his anxiety from 0 to 10. Remember that 0 represents no anxiety, a calm relaxed state that is alert and highly functioning. A 10 is the worst panic ever, generally as intense as one of your child's first panic attacks, when the symptoms were new and overwhelming.

It's more difficult to teach a child to describe the subtle intermediate numbers that measure anxiety. An essential step in breaking the Dragon's hold on your child is recognizing that anxiety is not an all-or-nothing state. Your child will likely have trouble understanding that anxiety is measured on a continuum. Work on creating an analogy or an explanation that makes sense for your child. Preschool-age children and those who have difficulty with numbers do better with small, medium, or big Dragons, than with using numbers like 6 that may be out of their developmental framework. Again, you know your child. Play to your child's strength. Does she like stuffed animals or stickers? Invest in three different sizes of Dragons, and show her that the fear can be big, medium, or small. Does she enjoy making graphs in school? Try using this knowledge to set up colorful graphs of anxiety levels.

The best way to take charge of anxiety is to keep a Journal. We will give you many ideas on how to use this Journal, but now is the

I am a Journal note, and I have advice for you in the 5 Steps of Part Two. A Journal can be a spiral or loose-leaf notebook or it can be kept on a computer. Pick a Journal and get it out *now*, before you go any further.

time to start one for your child. Begin by deciding whether this will be a Journal you keep of your child, for your child, or with your child. Remember, this is a Journal to work on reducing the power of the anxiety Dragon in your child's life, not a "Dear Diary"–type of book from which you will be excluded. It's fine for your child to have a separate diary, but this particular Journal will be a joint effort. Choosing who will take the lead as writer may take a while. You can always go back and change your arrangement later. For example, we worked with a thirteen-year-old who had a severe obsessive-compulsive disorder. She was scared to keep the Journal herself, because writing in it would have meant touching the Journal. Initially, her mother and her therapist wrote in the Journal for her. In sessions, the therapist wrote down techniques to try or therapy homework assignments to practice. Her mother wrote about the troubles and triumphs at home. After four sessions, this girl could touch the Journal and proudly took over the job of scribe. She kept the first part of the book as a reminder of how far she had come.

I can really terrify a child with high levels of fear—8, 9, and 10 are my favorites! Plus, I get to bug you, too, because it's so hard for you to watch your child suffer. I'm a trickster! (I hope you and your child don't figure out that even those high levels of anxiety can't actually harm your child!)

Ben was able to write in his own Journal, but Kurt, in Chapter 1, had a learning disability and couldn't keep the Journal himself. Neither learning disabilities nor physical handicaps should prevent a child from achieving full recovery. Some antianxiety techniques may have to be modified for certain kids. Kurt couldn't learn by writing in his Journal, but he could read about his accomplishments and his plans in the Journal. Some kids have a physical challenge, like asthma, food allergies, or a birth defect, that keeps them from doing things other kids take for granted. This is quite different from being limited by fear and anxiety. A child with asthma, for example, can keep track with a peak flow meter of how much difficulty he has breathing while playing a sport and can use medication if he needs it. Fear of having an asthma attack should not stop a child from doing something he wants to do, as long as his doctor says it is medically appropriate. For example, if he wants to jump into piles of hay at an autumn farm festival, that isn't likely to be good for his asthma! But jumping into a swimming pool might be fine.

A kid with attention deficit hyperactivity disorder may have trouble prioritizing homework and concentrating while doing assignments. This doesn't mean that he should be scared of homework or of learning, but rather that a tutor, medication, or another accommodation should be used to help the child learn to the best of his ability.

These first Journal entries give you a chance to record a baseline for your child's anxiety problem. When scientists do research, they start with a baseline for their measurements, to refer back to, in order to see changes that occur over time. From here on, as you and your child work with the Dragon and the Wizard, you can always look back on this time period and mark whether your child is better or worse than he was at the beginning.

In Chapter 8, Morgan's story of PTSD, her mother never had any trouble with anxiety. Her parents had divorced when she was a baby, though, so little was known about her paternal family history of anxiety or any other mental health problems. You will recall that anxiety can be a symptom of a more difficult to treat mental health problem in a child. This can be a frightening prospect for a parent, especially when the biological history is unknown. Because anxiety occurs at an earlier age than do other mental health problems and

can exist along with ADHD or depression, the simple steps out-
lined in this book might not help resolve your child's problem. Yet,
even if the techniques don't provide a total cure, you will have a
good record of what did and didn't work as you continue your
efforts to help your child.

## Assessing Whether Your Child Has an Anxiety Problem

|  | *Mild Problem* | *Moderate Problem* | *Severe Problem* |
|---|---|---|---|
| How long has this problem been present? | A few days. | A few weeks. | Six months or more. |
| How much suffering does your child have from this problem? | He does not seem distressed much of the time, or he is quite distressed for a short time and then is fairly easily calmed. | He seems distressed quite a bit but still has times when he is calm and happy. | He seems quite distressed most of the time and hardly ever experiences calm periods. |
| How much disability does this problem cause, with respect to your child's education and social life? | He does not miss school because of this problem. He has a normal extracurricular schedule in comparison to his peers. | He misses some school due to this problem and does not participate in some extracurricular activities or go to parties and play dates. | He has missed so much school that placement for next year is a dilemma. He does not have many friends and is socially isolated. |

Start each day by recording a few fear levels for your child. Perhaps you could casually check in with your child three times a day
to find out what fear levels she feels at that moment. Or have set
times each day when she writes in her Journal. Early Journal entries
will look something like this:

| | | | How Long Did |
|---|---|---|---|
| Time | Situation | Anxiety Level | the Anxiety Last? |
| 8 A.M. | Eating breakfast | 4 | 10 minutes |
| 1 P.M. | P.E. | 6 | 20 minutes |
| 9 P.M. | Bed | 6 | 5 minutes |

**Date: Friday**

Notice what makes the anxiety level go up and what makes it go down. Does your child seem to prime herself for fear in the morning? Does the level of anxiety often go up when she is in an unfamiliar place or when she feels alone? Or when she fears embarrassment or fears that she may become more afraid?

Noticing fear levels is a wonderful Wizard trick to help your child take control of anxiety. Just by noticing the anxiety, your child will learn that there are predictable times and places she has trouble with, and that will help both of you focus on how to make them better. More Wizard magic will come when your child notices that most of the time she doesn't feel anxiety! This is a crucial point. When you focus all of your energy on fear, you forget that most of the time you aren't afraid. Be sure to catch your child being unafraid, at a level of 0. Record these moments in the Journal. These two simple Wizard truths about anxiety will make a big difference in your child's life.

A third Wizard trick is to realize that fear, though sometimes intense, always goes away. Anxiety doesn't go up forever and doesn't last forever. These three simple Wizard observations help tremendously in understanding and being less fearful of the physical symptoms of anxiety. Your child's anxiety goes down when he waits and doesn't flee from the fearful situation. Fear goes down all on its own if he doesn't run away from what scares him. His fear will also drop to lower levels if he talks to you about it, as long as you respond calmly and reassuringly. Remind him that his fear goes down if he doesn't fear it and if he accurately observes it, as a scientist would check the temperature or the water level in a river.

Three of my best Wizard techniques:

1. Notice patterns in anxiety as it rises and falls.
2. Recognize that your child's anxiety level is 0 much of the time.
3. Appreciate that fear levels always come down.

Anxiety levels change moment to moment; they rarely stay the same for even a minute at a time. Study your child's anxiety level. You will become quite good at judging his fear levels. In our office, we are generally able to gauge a child's anxiety level from just a few minutes of talking. Low levels of anxiety are characterized by his being able to talk and play normally. A kid can play a good game of cards with Level 3 anxiety and will sit in a semirelaxed state while doing so. At Level 6, however, the cards are difficult to concentrate on, and the kid is likely to make mistakes, as his anxious feelings distract him, moment to moment. He may be able to stay seated while he plays but will probably be perched on the edge of his chair. At Level 8 anxiety, either a kid is rigid, with muscles clenched, as he pants or gasps for air, or else he is pacing with distress and noisy. It simply isn't possible to play even an easy game of cards at this level of anxiety, because the physical symptoms are so distracting.

My ability to scare your child is like a magic trick with mirrors. If I can keep her focused on my commands, she will stay under my control. If she finds fun things to do in life and doesn't pay attention to my tricks, I can't scare her and my thrills are over.

Difficult as it is to see your child in distress during a high level of anxiety, please remember that the Dragon can't do anything to your child except make him feel afraid. Be sure to point this out to your child. This is one secret the Dragon is most afraid that you'll discover. Once you know the Dragon can't hurt your child by making him behave strangely, become ill, or pass out, then the Dragon loses most of its power over him.

## Two Anxiety Inventories

We have developed two inventories that will help you evaluate your child's anxiety problem. The first is the Anxiety Inventory, sixteen questions that you can answer with your child. Each item is rated from 0, for no problem, to 3, for an extremely serious problem. Begin by rating the general level of your child's anxiety problem during the prior week. You will want to make many copies of this inventory or score it on separate pieces of paper, because it's helpful to repeat the inventory weekly when you begin the Anxiety Cure. After a few months you can fill out this inventory only monthly, unless there is a dramatic change in your child's anxiety. In that case, fill it out weekly or even daily. Keep the results of your Anxiety Inventories for future reference. You'll be surprised at how much your child's scores go down over time. That's the good news. The bad news is that even as your child gets better, there will be weeks when the anxiety is more active. At those times, your child's scores will rise temporarily. Don't let those setbacks discourage either of you. It's all part of the process of getting well.

The second inventory we ask you to complete is the Specific Anxiety Inventory. Here you'll find a short description of each of the six core anxiety disorders. (For a full description of these six anxiety disorders, review Chapter 2.) Using this inventory, check the one or ones that more or less apply to your child, even if you don't think your child fits the full, official diagnosis. Put a 1 in the diagnostic category that is the most severe now and a 2 in the category that is next-most severe, numbering as many of the six anxiety disorders as apply to your child. Circle the one diagnostic category that occurred first in your child's life.

When asking yourself whether your child has an anxiety problem, consider three factors. The first is how long the problem has lasted. Many childhood worries and fears are brief and of little significance. If, in contrast to this transience, your child's anxiety

**Anxiety Inventory**

May be filled out by an adult for a child.

---

0 = does not describe me      2 = describes me mostly

1 = describes me somewhat    3 = describes me completely

1. I am a tense person.                                    0 1 2 3

2. I worry more than most people do.                       0 1 2 3

3. I have a hard time relaxing.                            0 1 2 3

4. I have unexpected panic attacks.                        0 1 2 3

5. I avoid particular situations, things, or
   places because of extreme fear.                         0 1 2 3

6. When I'm anxious, I have physical
   symptoms.                                               0 1 2 3

7. I find excuses not to do things because
   of my anxiety.                                          0 1 2 3

8. I'm embarrassed by the things I can or
   cannot do because of anxiety.                           0 1 2 3

9. I have horrible thoughts that I cannot
   stop.                                                   0 1 2 3

10. I have to do things over and over
    because of fear or worry.                              0 1 2 3

11. I'm usually shy and uncomfortable at
    times when other people are not.                       0 1 2 3

12. My work suffers or sometimes I cannot
    work because of my anxiety.                            0 1 2 3

13. My family or friends notice that
    I'm anxious.                                           0 1 2 3

14. My family or friends find my anxiety
    upsetting.                                             0 1 2 3

15. I depend on my family or friends to do
    things because of my anxiety.                          0 1 2 3

16. I have lost contact with my family or
    friends because of my anxiety.                         0 1 2 3

## Specific Anxiety Disorder Inventory

| *Check if this is a possible problem and rank problems as most to least distressing* | *Anxiety Symptoms* | *Approximate date (day, month, year) when symptoms started* |
| --- | --- | --- |
| | Agoraphobia/Panic Disorder—My child has extreme anxiety or panic attacks when he is away from a safe person or a safe place. My child experiences panic attacks out of the blue. | |
| | Specific Phobia—My child has extreme anxiety or panic attacks when she is in specific situations, such as closed places, high places, or when flying, or about specific things, such as thunderstorms, animals, or insects. | |
| | Social Anxiety Disorder—My child has severe anxiety about public speaking, avoids public speaking, or is shy and uncomfortable in social situations like school or at a party. My child has an extreme fear of embarrassment. | |
| | Generalized Anxiety Disorder—My child worries about many things. Anxiety causes her significant distress or disability. These worries are not about one specific problem or about other anxiety disorders, such as worries about cleanliness or having a panic attack. | |
| | Obsessive-Compulsive Disorder—My child has intrusive, repugnant, unwanted thoughts (obsessions) and performs rituals (compulsions) like excessive hand washing, magical touching, or checking to try to reduce his fears of those terrible thoughts. | |
| | Posttraumatic Stress Disorder—My child had a severe trauma in his life and afterward developed nightmares and flashbacks, in which he seems to relive the terrible experience. My child has anxiety and depression. | |

persists for months or years, it is likely to be a significant problem. Second, consider how upset your child is as a result of the problem. Anxiety problems produce a high level of distress because anxiety is very painful. Third, look at the limitations imposed on your child. Anxiety problems can severely handicap a child.

Even more than with adults, the Dragon can appear in different ways in various settings with children. It can be a terrible shock after working hard to overcome one type of problem only to have the Dragon show up in another form. Remember, it's often difficult to narrow down which diagnostic category best fits a child because the anxiety symptoms can shift quickly over a short period of time. That's why it makes sense to learn the many ways that anxiety can be felt and explained. Behavior, feelings, words, and situations, all are possible arenas for anxiety. Since there is no way to predict what will happen to children who have anxiety, it's important to focus on today's problems but also to understand the difficulties tomorrow could bring.

What about you and the other members of your family? Do you have an anxiety problem? Do other members of your family? It will help everyone if you all openly discuss this issue. You may be surprised by what you discover. Anxiety problems are family problems. Getting well is an opportunity for the whole family. If adults in your family need help with an anxiety problem, you may want to read our book *The Anxiety Cure*. It contains more specific

Anxiety symptoms are common in other mental health problems. While 13 percent of children have a diagnosable anxiety disorder, 6.2 percent have a mood disorder, and 10.3 percent have a disruptive disorder. Often these diagnoses overlap in a child. A child with more than one mental health problem will benefit from seeing a therapist, taking medication, and receiving a clear message from his parents about what is expected of him. (U.S. Department of Health and Human Services. *Mental Health: A Report of the Surgeon General*, 1999) techniques and information about problems faced by anxious adults, such as handling anxiety at work and dealing with anxiety in the elderly.

## Anxious Children Can Help Anxious Adults

Children of all ages are less likely than adults to rationalize their anxiety problems. They tend to express anxiety through behavior, rather than through words. Children are also less likely than adults to excuse their anxiety problems. All of this makes it easier for kids to recover because the cure has everything to do with their actions. In many families, the child's confrontation with the Dragon empowers a parent or a sibling to tackle a long-neglected anxiety problem. Anxious children are eager to help adults and siblings who also suffer from anxiety. Truly, it is said, "The best way to learn anything is to teach it." Your child will better understand what it takes for him to get well by helping you or someone else in your family overcome an anxiety problem.

## Respect the Dragon

We encourage families not to fight the Dragon. Don't disrespect it. We want you to tame it. That means talking to it like this:

"Hi, Dragon. We understand you now a lot better than we did before. Come along with us. Right now, we want to do a few things. You're welcome to come with us."

The Dragon won't be satisfied with this. It will growl and snort and blow fiery breath at your child. It wants your child to feed it with fear. Help your child say:

"No, Dragon, I don't fear you anymore. I respect you, but I don't fear you."

Once the Dragon believes this—and it will take a while for the Dragon to be convinced that your child means what he says—the Dragon will shrink because it can eat only your child's fear. It will come to visit your child less often.

Remember this about the Dragon, though. It often comes back, sometimes taking you and your child by surprise after it's been gone a long time. But whenever the Dragon comes back, whether it's been gone a short or a long time, just say, "Hello, Mr. Dragon, where have you been all this time? We knew you would come back because we read in a book that this is how Dragons work. So, welcome back. We're a busy family, so just tag along as much as you want to."

Sometimes I can find experiences from your child's past that were especially painful and can use them to make a new fear. These repeating patterns of painful memories or even situations are a neat trick of mine. I can keep you or your child stuck in horrendous anxiety for years unless you find a way to untwist your thinking. You may need a therapist or a self-help group to do that.

When you say this, the Dragon again loses interest in your child. When it surprises you both and your child begins to fear it again, the Dragon is very happy. It quickly grows larger and larger until you and your child remember what you have learned in this book and stop feeding it with fear.

## Set Initial Goals for Your Child

When your child was born, you had hopes and dreams for his future. Some of these desires were based on things you had as a child; some might have been based on what you didn't have as a child. Having a child gives us a wonderful opportunity to do things the way we wish we had experienced them ourselves. Reflecting on what you wished for is important. Take a moment to think about your dreams as you anticipated the arrival of your child, whether he is your biological child or not. These dreams are based on an imaginary idea of the child, before you know him, but they can subtly color your expectations as he grows.

Jacqueline, whose socialite mother had spent little time with her when she was young, was a stay-at-home mother who never traveled away from her three children. She had hoped to have four children but had experienced repeated miscarriages during the ten years between the birth of her second and third child. Her first two children were boys, and by the time she had her youngest, a girl, she was forty-two and knew it was unlikely that she would have any more children. This final child was the recipient of Jacqueline's dreams even before being born. Her nursery was a pink wonderland, and she and her mother were never separated. When Jacqueline's daughter, Tammy, was thirteen years old, her school planned an overnight field trip, and Jacqueline could not attend, because she had to be with her husband to receive an important award. Jacqueline and Tammy were devastated at being separated overnight. They came into our office hoping to get a doctor's note that would excuse Tammy from the trip. Instead, we asked Jacqueline to come in for several individual sessions to talk about this extraordinarily close relationship between her and her daughter. Jacqueline considered this closeness a wonderful blessing, almost a redemption for the rejection she had felt from her own mother as a child. We helped Jacqueline see that the close relationship was terrific but also created in each of them the fear that they couldn't function independently. We pointed out that her sons had done well with less attention and that nonetheless she felt quite close to them as well. For the first trial separation, we suggested that Tammy have dinner at a friend's house and go to a movie without her mother. Jacqueline missed Tammy terribly during this practice separation and recalled with nostalgia the years that they had been together all the time. The next practice separation we made plans for Jacqueline, as well as for Tammy, and Jacqueline was surprised that she actually had fun being the substitute in a tennis doubles game one evening.

Before Jacqueline thought about this problem in light of her own dreams, her goals for Tammy were different from those we came up with together. Although the goal of having a close relationship was wonderful, it didn't allow Tammy to grow in independence as a teenager and actually created separation phobias in both mother and daughter. Jacqueline's limited goal for Tammy didn't allow her daughter to grow.

In contrast, some parents come to the sad realization that their child's mental illness is more than an anxiety disorder and that the treatment path is longer and more complex. Amanda came in to talk about John's anxiety in school. This anxiety, however, was diagnosed as being caused by John's paranoid thoughts that everyone was after him, which led him to cower in the bathroom, crying for help against beings no one else could see. This was a serous problem that required hospitalization. The suggestions in our book can be useful in a situation like this, but only with the guidance of therapists and psychiatrists.

> Self-confidence comes from setting a goal—even a small goal like confronting one's fears—and then attaining that goal by sustained hard work. This process can give your child confidence to move on to new goals. Many adults make the mistake of thinking that the anxious child would be more independent if he were more self-confident. Actually, it works the other way around. Your child's self-confidence will increase only when he takes small but persistent steps toward becoming more independent in his actions and, most important, in his thinking. That means facing and accepting the pain of anxiety and living a "normal life," despite his anxious feelings. Running away from fear lowers self-esteem and weakens his ability to overcome the Dragon's powers. Moving toward the source of fear, even in small steps, with your encouragement and support, builds your child's self-confidence and loosens the Dragon's grip on him.

If your child has a food allergy, a physical handicap, or a major mental health illness, please keep these limitations in mind as you set goals for his future. Although it isn't helpful to a child to set goals too low, it's also unfair to expect him to do things that are simply impossible. Setting realistic goals may be hard for you to do. To get beyond your own perspective, ask a trusted friend for help.

Your child may surprise you by exceeding your expectations. Celebrate this achievement, and move on to higher goals. We have seen this scenario far more often with children than we have seen the reverse. Think about school, home life, and extracurricular activities when you set goals for his future.

|  | *Current Functioning* | *Goals for the Future* |
|---|---|---|
| Home |  |  |
| School |  |  |
| Extracurricular Activities |  |  |

When setting goals for the present, consider your child's age. Clearly, an appropriate goal for a three-year-old is different from that for a thirteen-year-old! Finding a balance between independence and safety is hard for parents. Think about how your dreams for your child play into this evaluation. What types of freedoms and responsibilities did you have when you were his age? What are your spouse's memories of this age? In general, you want your child to be safe, but not at the cost of learning independence and self-confidence. Your fears may limit the amount of freedom you allow your child, and his fears may limit the degree of freedom he can tolerate. Self-confidence will come from realizing that he can solve a problem on his own. Think of safe ways you can let your child feel independent. How about doing household chores, like caring for a pet or keeping an eye on a younger sibling? Or learning to do the wash or cook dinner? These tasks can all be done safely, in an-age appropriate way, and can lead to increased self-confidence.

**Goal Chart**

|  | *Predicted Anxiety: If your child did this today* | *Actual Anxiety: When your child accomplishes this goal* |
|---|---|---|
| 1. |  |  |
| 2. |  |  |
| 3. |  |  |
| 4. |  |  |

Setting goals is hard, yet it's also the most important part of an anxiety cure. Again and again, we have seen that working to overcome an anxiety problem ends up improving the child's or the entire family's ability to function. Think about goals for your child not in the context of your past dreams but as attainable possibilities for your child and your family. Set a hierarchy of goals, some that will be easy to achieve, and others that seem impossible at this point. For each goal, come up with ideas that will help you both achieve them. The fact that you're reading this book means that you would like to make some changes. Keep an open mind, so that you'll be receptive to new ideas that might lead to progress. Changing isn't easy, but the outcome can be amazing and wonderful.

## Homework for Step 1

1. Start your Journal! Write or have your child write his name, age, and today's date. One boy started his Journal with this entry:

   "About Me"
   I go to North Farms School. My name is Jim. I'm almost 8. My best friends are Sam and Adam. The End.

2. Write or have your child write the answers to these questions about his anxiety Dragon.
   - What are you afraid of?
   - When did your fear start?
   - What has helped you feel better?
   - Do you feel the fear now? How much, 0 to10?
   - Right now, how do you feel? Very happy / happy / scared / sad / angry / don't know.
   - Are you scared a lot?
   - What is one thing you wish you were not scared of?
   - What is one time when you felt that being scared helped you stay safe?
   - Who can you count on to help when you are scared?

3. Set up your child's anxiety Journal. Describe your child's level of fear daily, rating how scared he is from 0, no fear, to 10, the worst possible fear.

4. Record ten practical goals for getting better from anxiety. List specific things for your child to do, like sleeping over at a friend's house or reading a book for fifteen minutes without ritualized counting. Some of these goals should be easy and some harder. Your child will not do them all at once, and not sooner than she is ready to. These goals will help you and your child pick directions for your work in the next chapters.

5. Have your child rate each goal from 0 to 10, as if she had to do that task today. This will help you sort out which homework to start with in the next chapter.

| Date | Practice Plan | Anticipated Anxiety Level | Actual Anxiety Level | Time Spent Practicing | Wizard Magic Used |
|------|---------------|---------------------------|----------------------|-----------------------|-------------------|
|      |               |                           |                      |                       |                   |
|      |               |                           |                      |                       |                   |

### Action Steps

- It can be painful to see how far your child has to go before reaching the goals you've set for him, but at least all of your activities will work toward achieving those goals.
- Allow room to reconsider certain goals, if his interest or anxiety changes over time.
- Remind yourself and your child that high levels of anxiety are distressing but not dangerous. Even severe anxiety goes away with the passage of time.

CHAPTER 6

# Step 2

*Julie's Story—Shrink the Dragon with*
*Practice and Cognitive Restructuring*

Julie was a five year old, with a mop of curly hair and big brown eyes. She wasn't afraid of anyone or anything—except for getting shots or having blood taken by a doctor or a nurse. At her last medical check-up, Julie had to have three shots to get ready for school. She yelled and cried, embarrassing both her mom and herself. Her mom helped the nurse hold Julie down while the doctor gave her the shots. Julie was angry for weeks about that experience. She said that she would rather die than get another shot. In Julie's family, everyone had to get tested for high cholesterol, which meant that Julie had to have blood drawn from her arm. Before this procedure, the doctor talked to her mom about helping Julie be less afraid. The doctor didn't want Julie to be so upset about something that is easy for most children. Julie knew that the rest of her family had already taken the blood test. She knew that giving blood was not a big deal to anyone else in her family. No one likes to get a shot or get blood drawn—or, for that matter, to get stitches for a cut—but Julie's feelings were more extreme than other children's. She was terrified of needles. She didn't have panic attacks. She wasn't afraid to speak up in class. In fact if she didn't have to think about shots, she was never anxious or worried. But her fear of needles was a very big problem.

Julie's mom came in to see us. We explained how the Dragon worked and that Julie's fears and powerful feelings were very real to her. We also said that we could teach Julie the Wizard's techniques to tame the Dragon. When we later met with Julie and her mom, Julie was glad that we weren't going to give her any shots. We told her about the Dragon and why she was so much more afraid of shots than the rest of her family was. We said, "The more scared you are of something, the more that thing hurts. The more you can relax and calm yourself, the less it hurts. This is good to know about all kinds of painful experiences." Julie said that even though she never wanted any more shots, she knew that she would eventually have to get one, so she wanted to become less afraid so that the shots would hurt less.

We helped Julie by teaching her this Wizard technique. Julie actually had a lot of control over what happened, even though she didn't realize it. The Dragon wanted her to feel helpless, but she really wasn't. For example, she could choose which arm would get the shot. She could count from the moment the needle pricked her skin, "One, two, three, four . . . ," to find out how long it actually took to get a shot. Counting works well for having blood drawn, too. We told Julie that she'd be surprised at how quickly both procedures were over. Even if for a few seconds she hurt a medium amount from the needle, that brief pain surely wasn't worth spending days being upset before and after a shot!

Another Wizard technique, learning more about an actual situation she feared, helped Julie a lot. We showed her the rest of the equipment that nurses use to give shots, so that Julie could handle it. We gave her a tourniquet to put on her arm. We showed her the syringe—without a needle on it. She liked learning about the vacuum in the tubes used to collect the blood sample. With no fear of having a shot at that moment, Julie was interested in learning what the instruments were and how the nurses used them.

Julie and her mother went home to practice with the lab equipment on Julie's collection of stuffed animals. They practiced counting and relaxing. The next day Julie's mom called us to report that Julie was now ready to get her blood drawn. Julie knew that the Wizard would help her when she took charge herself. That's why

Julie chose the day for blood to be drawn. She and her mom went to the doctor's office, and Julie had her blood taken with no problem. She chatted with the nurse and identified all of the equipment the nurse used. Julie's mother was amazed, and Julie was very proud of herself. In fact, her whole family was proud. Now Julie was a girl who truly feared nothing. She was especially proud of working hard to overcome her fear. Her hard work paid off with good results, like taming that anxiety Dragon in her head. Julie and her mom talked about how the Dragon might show up again—because of needles or something else—and how Julie could use her Wizard magic if that happened.

> If you are keeping a Journal for a child who cannot yet read, use symbols or stickers to help him participate in filling out the daily logs.

## Step 2: Tame the Dragon

Your child can tame the Dragon by strengthening her own mind and by practicing the very things that the Dragon makes her think she should avoid. This is usually tough, especially at first. It's like learning a new sport or a card game. It can be hard to keep track of all the tricks of the game, but if your child keeps trying to shrink the Dragon, she'll get better each time she practices. Her mind will be stronger, more able to handle her fears—the Dragon's attacks. This skill will help her throughout her entire life. You can also help by teaching her about the Dragon and the scale to measure anxiety.

> Kids can recover remarkably fast from an anxiety problem if they use my magic. Parents may be shocked that a problem they have worked around and been concerned with for so long can vanish almost overnight. My magic is strong. It works. Just keep track in your Journal of how I can help, in case that nasty Dragon returns.

Mostly, however, you support your child by believing in her ability to do this practice. You must feel calm yourself, knowing that even if her anxiety goes up, the practice is useful. Anxiety, no matter how severe, will not harm your child.

Even if your child uses no other Wizard trick, be sure she understands the importance of practicing what she fears. She'll find that it's not possible to continue to fear the Dragon after she has practiced any anxiety-causing situation enough times.

When your child runs away from her fear, the fear runs after her and grows larger and stronger. When she turns and faces her fear, the fear backs off. It's just like learning to ride a bike or play a game or learning math or how to write—it seems impossible at first, but with lots of practice it becomes easy. Remember when you held the bike for your child and ran up and down the street behind her? You played "Go Fish" a million times until it became second nature for her. That's what we want you to do now—help your child understand so that she can master these techniques. You can help her take back control of her life from the scary anxiety Dragon.

The intense emotion your child feels when anxiety symptoms appear reinforces the memory links in her brain that keep the anxiety coming back again and again. She needs to learn not to respond to anxiety with intense, negative emotion, in order to break this link. Then the pattern is not emotion paired with anxiety but, rather, simple anxiety, which her brain will experience without added emotion for only a few minutes. (Bremmer and Charney. *Textbook of Anxiety Disorders* [Washington, D.C.: American Psychiatric Publishing, Inc., 2002])

There are two basic ways to deal with the Dragon: With your help, your child must change her thoughts first and change her actions second. This approach, under the guidance of a therapist, is called cognitive-behavioral therapy, or CBT for short. Cognitively, your child will change her thoughts about the Dragon, and behaviorally, she will change what she does when the Dragon shows up. Research shows that combining changes in thoughts and behavior is a powerful way to overcome anxiety. Your Journal will reveal over time that your child really has changed how she thinks and acts. Most people don't intuitively understand how they can change the way they think, much less help their child change the way she thinks.

### Five Steps to Tame the Dragon

| Reminder Word | Explanation of this step. |
|---|---|
| Recognize | Recognize anxiety for what it is and let your child know that this is a Dragon fear. |
| Remind | Remind yourself and your child that she is not in danger. |
| Calm | Calm yourself and help your child find ways to calm herself. |
| Ally | Ally yourself with your child and against the Dragon. |
| Notice | Notice when anxiety fades. Praise your child later for her progress. |

By identifying her son's overwhelming feeling not as a real problem (of paper being stuck in his mouth) but as a Dragon fear, the mother in Chapter 3 changed the topic of conversation. This put the emphasis squarely where it belonged, on solving the problem of that irrational fear. The child, of course, felt in danger, because his feeling of anxiety was so strong. Nevertheless, when his mom reminded him that even though anxiety feels dangerous, it isn't really dangerous, he felt safer. Then he was able to do the next step on his own, calming himself by taking a deep breath, because he had practiced this many times. Finally, both mother and son were able to get mad that the dratted Dragon had prevented their enjoying the family party. By directing her anger at the Dragon, the mother was able to refrain from getting mad at her son. She knew he didn't want to misbehave, but he felt compelled by the anxiety to do so. The Dragon made him do it! Best of all, she noticed how quickly he recovered from this severe anxiety. At that moment of shared triumph, she made a mental note to congratulate him later.

> Twisting and wiggling serpent Dragons; evil, fire-spitting Dragons; kindly, protective Dragons that bring good luck—there are many kinds of Dragons from all around the world.
> —*BEHOLD . . . THE DRAGONS!* GAIL GIBBONS
> (HONG KONG: MORROW JUNIOR BOOKS, 1999)

When most people, both kids and adults, start to work on their anxiety problem, they have a hard time understanding that they can change how they act and think, and that this will change how they feel. We usually don't think about thinking. It can seem daunting for parents to try to understand how their child thinks. So much of a parent's focus is on the bothersome behavioral manifestations of the anxiety problem. Here's an example of how a kid's anxious thoughts work. Imagine a child who has to do a big project for school. He sits down to start work on it. Immediately, he worries that he won't be able to do a good job or won't finish it on time. The boy hears an inner message that says, "This project is too hard for me. I can't do it." Then he feels even worse! He feels so bad that he puts off even starting the project. The boy's anxious inner thoughts lead him to procrastinate, which is the behavior that parents finally notice.

Now imagine a different scenario. The boy is back at the stage where he just sat down to start the project. He feels worried and says to himself, "This is a big project, I need to figure out how to do it one step at a time. Let me start with a really small step, like

I do a good job of scaring people before medical procedures. Even that word *procedure* can be a really scary place to start. All that fear before the procedure makes children suffer much more than if they just had the shot or the stitches or whatever, without worrying about it beforehand. Take away the worry, and the pain of the procedure is gone before you know it! But worry in anticipation of something can be powerful and can last a long time.

writing my name on a piece of paper." He finds many separate steps to doing this big project. It's easier to complete just one tiny step at a time. This positive reframing of the frightening, overwhelming situation helps the boy gain confidence to start his work. That shrinks the anxiety Dragon. Parents can see only the resulting behavior: the kid doing his work! This inner dialogue is easier for older school-age kids and adolescents, but even younger children can understand that part of anxiety. At all ages, when children practice behavior that aims in a positive direction, toward the goal, it increases self-confidence. Avoidance always lowers self-confidence.

**The Project**

|            | Thought        | Action                        | Anxiety | Self-Esteem |
|------------|----------------|-------------------------------|---------|-------------|
| Dragon Way | I can't do this. | Delay starting.             | High    | Low         |
| Wizard Way | I need a plan. | Start working on small steps. | Low     | High        |

This example may reveal how thoughts and actions lead to anxious feelings, but you may still find it tough to figure out how to make this work with your child. Try setting up a chart like the previous one to record a situation in your child's Journal. There's nothing like a real-life example to make the process clearer. Let's say your first-grader has missed school all week because she had an unexplained stomach pain but didn't have a fever. She didn't throw up or have diarrhea. The pediatrician found nothing wrong. She didn't want you to leave her side this week while she was home from school. She cried hysterically every night, not wanting to be alone in her bedroom. The weekend before this behavior started, she had seen the movie *Harry Potter* with a good friend. She seemed cheerful when she came home but said the movie was too scary. Let's look at how a chart illustrates this problem.

### The Stomach Ache

|  | *Thought* | *Action* | *Anxiety* | *Self-Esteem* |
|---|---|---|---|---|
| Dragon Way | Monsters will get me. | Cling to mom. | High | Low |
| Wizard Way | It was just a movie. There is no such thing as Voldemort. | Go to school. | Low | High |

It's easy to imagine the distraught mother in this situation. She might feel guilty for letting her daughter go to the movie with a friend. She might be concerned that her daughter really was physically ill. She would worry about her daughter's missing so much school. She might also be unsure of what to say to friends and to the girl's teacher. The way to avoid all of this is by helping the child with a new thought: "It was just a movie; there is no such thing as Voldemort." Now, the child might still be afraid of monsters and might believe this new thought only a little bit. That's OK. Remember, we're just starting. If a child believes that the new thought *might* be true, there's room for the child to try it out. The new thought could even lead to her going back to school. School will certainly distract her and fill her head with enough thoughts to crowd out those about the movie she saw.

Remember, one of the best ways for your child to get through an anxious situation is to think about a task and not about her fear. This means distracting herself from whatever the Dragon is making her feel. The Dragon is a jealous master and wants your child to think only of it. The more your child thinks about the Dragon,

Counting how long it takes to get through a dreaded experience works well in lots of disturbing situations. With a child who has a phobia of bridges or tunnels, for example, make a game out of guessing how long it will take to go over the bridge or through the tunnel, and count the time together. Counting also provides a way to time the actual event, as opposed to focusing on the anticipatory anxiety, which is where most of the suffering occurs.

the more your child fears it. This means the Dragon is fat and happy. If your child refocuses her attention, for example, by thinking up a practical plan to accomplish a big project, she can stop herself from feeding the Dragon. In the previous example, getting back to school is the distraction from the feelings of anxiety. This week, concentrate on having your child practice some distracting skills. When she is anxious, remind her to focus on other work, get up and move, play with a friend or a pet, talk on the phone, or think of a joke. We use the word *distracting*, but it's really the Dragon that is "distracting," because anxiety distracts your child from important experiences in life. What we call "distraction" amounts to replacing the Dragon's unwanted distraction with real life.

The changes that your child puts into place through her new non-frightened actions and thoughts will change her brain chemistry. Research shows that people with OCD who successfully complete treatment in cognitive-behavioral therapy actually have brains that function like those of normal people. The "cured" brain is distinctly different from the frightened, abnormal brain. (Schwartz, et al. *Archives of General Psychiatry*, vol. 53 [1996]: 109–113)

The behavioral part of recovering from an anxiety problem means that your child needs to practice doing the very things that make her anxious. This will show the Dragon that she isn't afraid of it, even if it makes her feel bad. Remind your child that the Dragon can't hurt her. Record a series of simple, easy goals for her. These goals will help you chart your child's progress. They don't have to be hard goals. In fact, your child will enjoy looking back on some of the easy goals, after she has found new ways to handle the anxiety-provoking situations for herself.

> Even with all my tricks, I can't make your child feel scared of things she is used to doing. Drat! Only things that she doesn't often do can be scary, which is why I try to keep her in my prison and away from doing normal, healthy activities.

Try to find specific goals, like going to school today, or going to the library bathroom with the door closed. These goals should be clear, so that you and your child will know whether she has reached them. Don't make her feelings the goal. For example, don't set as a goal "I will feel less anxious when I ride an escalator." The goal should be, "I will ride the escalator at the shopping mall." If it's too hard for your child to even think about setting a goal, even a small one, you may need a therapist to help with this or a doctor to prescribe an antianxiety medication to help your child while she confronts her fears.

## Homework for Step 2

1. Set up a chart like the one for the Project, and find a new thought and a new action to help with one of your child's anxious situations.
2. Set up a new practice chart for your child to use instead of her anxiety Journal. You will no longer merely watch your child's anxiety; now you will seek anxiety-provoking situations that provide a chance to practice. Set up a four-column anxiety practice Journal like the following one.

## Weekly Practice Chart

*Your Child's Goal for This Week:* _____

| Date | Practice Activity | Predicted Anxiety* | Actual Anxiety* |
|------|-------------------|--------------------|-----------------|
|      |                   |                    |                 |
|      |                   |                    |                 |
|      |                   |                    |                 |

*Rate 0–10

3. Record two situations where your child will practice new thoughts and actions during the next seven days. Be sure that they are situations that will cause your child anxiety that ranges from a Level 2 to a Level 5.

> Reality is very powerful in combating the Dragon. I don't ask you to tell your child that things are great when they don't feel good to her at all. Rather, I want you to help her look at the facts. The Dragon cannot hurt your child. She is learning how to handle her anxiety problem. These powerful truths will banish the negative falsehoods that the Dragon tells your child.

### Action Steps

- Review your child's Journal for today and her practice plan for tomorrow. It is likely that she will find many more places and times to practice than you would expect.
- Encourage her to think about every moment of Dragon fear as an opportunity to make progress with help from the Wizard.

CHAPTER 7

# Step 3

*William's Story: Using Medication
and Relaxation*

William was twelve when we saw him. He liked to play with his
friends in the neighborhood after school. Usually, they played basketball, Monopoly, or card games. School was tough for William
that year because bad thoughts came to him over and over. He felt
like he absolutely had to do certain things just so. He had to touch
things in a certain way to keep them clean. He had to make a funny
noise that sounded like a little whistle when things got especially
bad. The kids teased William because of these peculiar actions and
sounds. Other children purposely knocked over William's books or
patted him on the back to upset him. He hated that. Then he would
whistle in that odd way because he was so upset. That made the
other kids laugh even harder.

These problems had started slowly the year before. William tried
not to tell his mom and dad about them because he couldn't understand them himself. One day, though, he had a crisis and had to tell
his mother.

He had been in physical education class at school, which was a
major problem for him anyway, because the kids had to sit on the
floor for roll call. William felt that sitting on the floor was unclean.
The crisis began when William saw a flag football teammate sneeze

115

onto his hand during the game. William and the kid had been in the middle of the game when this happened. As the game went on, William became convinced that he was being covered with germs from this kid's unwashed hands. The germs were carried on a ball they all used. After gym class, William washed his hands for half an hour. Even then, he couldn't open his locker or touch his books. He felt so dirty, he was afraid to walk into class and sit at his desk. He stood in the hall outside his locker, frozen in fear, holding his hands out in front of him. His teacher sent him to the nurse, who called his mother.

William came to see us the next day. He looked haunted as he held his hands straight out as if they were covered with mud. His hands looked fine to us. We explained to him and to his parents about the anxiety Dragon and how to label his fear from 0 to 10. We told William that he could find a Wizard in his mind to help him fight the Dragon, and that we would teach him some good Wizard tricks. This was all new information for William and his parents. At first, William had a hard time believing that other kids could have problems like his. We gave his parents a list of books about anxiety to read. We asked them to tell William about the other kids' stories in the books, because William couldn't imagine touching a book himself. He still felt contaminated from the sneeze during the football game the day before. William worked hard for two days with his parents, his therapist, and a psychiatrist, who prescribed him an antianxiety medication. Mostly, his own hard work made him well enough to go back to school.

After William understood his anxiety problems, he was determined to shrink his Dragon. When he felt able to touch his anxiety Journal, he kept it up to date and complete. He liked learning Wizard tricks. He practiced doing things that were a little hard and shrank his Dragon slowly, day after day. After about four weeks of working, William noticed that he was a lot better. Not only was he back in school, but he was also practicing things like touching the floor and then eating lunch without washing his hands. As a result of this work, the anxiety Dragon wasn't a big problem anymore.

However, his strange whistling remained a problem. The kids still teased him about it, even though he wasn't bothered now if his books were out of order or fell on the floor. William began to practice a new Wizard trick. His therapist recorded a relaxation tape that let William practice breathing slowly, instead of making that whistling noise. William liked doing this practice. It felt good to do it and was much easier than the practice he had done while shrinking his Dragon. After only a few days of practice, he stopped whistling when he got upset. The kids then stopped teasing him because it was no longer fun now that William didn't get upset and whistle. William began to make friends at school. He knew that the Dragon no longer had any power over him. He knew that he had taken control of his life back from that Dragon. Now he knew how the Dragon worked. He knew just how to shrink the Dragon whenever it tried to come back into his life.

## Step 3: Learning How to Use Medication and Relaxation

Medication and cognitive-behavioral therapy are both effective in treating anxiety disorders. This is a profoundly important point, because it illustrates that there is no separation between the mind and the body. The mind-body connectedness allows us to see anxiety as not purely psychological or biological, but as a biopsychosocial phenomenon. (Ellison et al. *Textbook of Anxiety Disorders* [Washington, D.C.: American Psychiatric Publishing, Inc., 2002])

Medication and relaxation may seem like strange companions, but they are both tools to help an anxious child reduce the power of the Dragon. Though we don't call medication itself a Wizard trick, we do say that using medication can be a Wizard trick.

An important Wizard trick to remember is that small victories against the Dragon are often more effective than huge bursts of effort. Be sure to praise yourself and your child for the hard work you both do every day!

Using medication and relaxation offers a direct way to tap into the complex physiological and psychological cycles that create and sustain anxiety. While experiencing anxiety, a child's body has inappropriately activated a fight-or-flight mechanism. The child's brain reads this heightened arousal as a sign that there really is an emergency. Interrupting this fight-or-flight arousal by using medication or by consciously relaxing and breathing deeply reminds the brain that there's no emergency; everything is fine. It shows the brain that the anxiety is a false alarm. Though relaxation alone won't solve your child's problem, learning to relax and breathe deeply will help him combat the fierce physical anxiety symptoms that the Dragon provokes. William's story, as well as many other children's stories in this book, shows how medication can be used to manage a crisis, long-term high levels of anxiety, or the anxiety that is generated by practicing certain behaviors.

Here's a good Wizard trick to use if a bully is teasing your child. Ask your child to pretend that he is writing a script for a sitcom. "What would the character playing you say to the bully who is bothering you?"

When we first talk about the importance of practicing deep breathing and relaxation, kids and parents usually look annoyed or at least a bit uncertain. What they are uncertain about is us and our understanding of their problem. They *are* certain that this won't work for them. Most people feel that this remedy is way too simple for them. They feel that breathing and relaxation would be a good solution for people who don't really have an anxiety problem but only think they do. Most people immediately worry that we aren't taking their very real anxiety problem seriously. We do take it seriously. Each individual who comes to us looking for help is suffering. Each of you reading this book is also struggling with a family anxiety problem. Breathing and relaxation are not trivial solutions. As with all of the advice we offer, of course, relaxation won't work for everyone—but it will help most anxious people.

> Add some color to your child's Journal. Make it an illustrated workbook. Ask her to draw a picture of the Dragon at an anxiety level of 10 and at a level of 1. If she likes to draw, she can draw the Dragon at every number from 1 to 10.

Breathing is something most people don't think about very often. Your child's body automatically takes air in and out of his body twenty-four hours a day. Consciously breathing deeply, however, can help your child's body relax and be less tense or on edge. With these relaxation exercises, your child will find that his mind and his body are his friends.

> You know your child well, and you're learning more about anxiety every day. Professionals have spent many years in school and in clinics, working to help children with anxiety problems. Don't be shy about combining your expertise with their knowledge. Your child needs help now, not after your years of study and hard work. If a therapist or a psychiatrist can become your teacher, take advantage of that expertise.

Medication can also help your child become friends with his body. Now that you have worked on the first two steps, recording how much and at what times your child has anxiety and setting practice goals, you may decide to talk to a therapist, a psychiatrist, or your child's pediatrician about trying medication to reduce anxiety. Remember, the techniques in this book will work well over time, but kids may need additional help from medication, especially when they start to practice doing things they are afraid of. If you are not in contact now with a health professional about your child, make a list of the pros and cons of seeing someone for help. Finding a referral to a therapist or a psychiatrist may be on your own list of homework for this week.

If your child is already using medication, it's vitally important to keep a careful record of the medications your child tries over time. Set up this chart in your child's Journal:

| Medication | Dates Taken | Dose | Side Effects? | Helpfulness |
|---|---|---|---|---|
|  |  |  |  |  |
|  |  |  |  |  |
|  |  |  |  |  |

In your child's Journal, review the anxiety your child has experienced. The anxiety may fall into two different categories: either your child has anxiety most of the time, at a low to moderate level, or your child may have short, sudden, and intense feelings of panic in certain situations or out of the blue and then may have little or no panic the rest of the time. A child may move from one category to another over time. William, at the beginning of this chapter, at first had obsessive thoughts and anxiety only intermittently. When he got worse, but before his anxiety crisis, he continually dwelled on worried thoughts. During the crisis, the anxiety was constant. Then, after he began using medication and had learned how to cope with his anxiety and shrink his Dragon, he had worried thoughts only occasionally. Notice that the relaxation helped William in this last situation. He had managed to shrink his

Dragon with medication, practice, and cognitive restructuring. When it came to the last part, coping with the unpredictable pattern of his whistling symptom, relaxation helped him the most.

Relaxation also works well for a child who has a low to moderate level of anxiety most of the time. If a child can make it a habit to practice relaxing or deep breathing three times a day for a week, he can drop his average anxiety level a few points on the 0 to 10 scale. This can make a dramatic difference in his feeling and functioning, because low levels become 0, and moderate levels, those that generally distract one from achieving a good level of functioning, become low levels.

A painful Dragon trick is to make you and your child focus on how far you still have to go in working toward a cure. I don't want you to look back at how far you have come. Instead, I want you to see only the long, long road ahead. I can make that road seem very long and lonely, can't I?

A child at a high level of anxiety—say, 8 to 10—or a child who has a tough time sitting still may have difficulty concentrating during the relaxation exercise or the travel imagery script. Start by working with your child on the breathing exercise. You'll need to breathe deeply yourself to show your child how to do it. This may

If you are undecided about whether your child needs medication or therapy, take an interim step at this point. Find a referral and call a mental health professional on the phone to establish availability and cost. Make your own judgment about whether the person sounds qualified and compatible with you. By getting professional help, you are avoiding the Dragon trap that says this would be admitting a major problem with your child. You are also giving yourself a future option, should your child's anxiety become worse.

benefit you, too. Having a child with an anxiety problem can be stressful for a parent. Relaxation and deep breathing can be a great way to release some of that tension.

Anxiety triggers and is triggered by the fight-or-flight response of imminent danger. The frightened body tenses; breathing becomes shallow and fast. That's how your body prepares for danger. When faced with anxiety, your mind becomes narrowly focused and you are hypervigilant. That's how your mind prepares for danger. In truly dangerous situations, it's a great help in mobilizing a quick response to fight or flee. But with an anxiety problem, the fight-or-flight response is a false alarm of danger. In this exercise you will reverse the signals from your body. By practicing relaxation, you create bodily effects opposite those of anxiety. Your breathing is deep and slow. Your mind is focused on your breathing, not on the Dragon. Just as anxiety triggers more anxiety, when your body reverses the signals to the brain, the brain changes. It is quieted. This is called "the relaxation response." It's built into your body and your brain. With practice, you and your child can harness the relaxation response to reverse the vicious cycle of anxiety begetting more anxiety. Mastering these relaxation techniques helps your child fear the Dragon less, which means feeding him less.

Begin to practice deep breathing without your child around, because you might feel silly when you start. You will need two books to practice breathing; midsized novels work well. Lie with your back on the floor. Place one book on your chest and one on your stomach. Take a big breath. If not instructed otherwise, most people will lift the book on their chest with this breath. Many people erroneously think that is where air fills us. Actually, as singers and athletes know, our body efficiently uses air that is pulled much lower into our lungs, by our diaphragm pushing down toward our gut. Take a breath again and this time try to make the lower book, the one on your stomach, rise.

Practice making your breath come in like a wave, traveling toward the lower part of your lungs and inflating them first, and then filling your chest with air. As you exhale, practice the reverse.

Wizard magic often looks deceptively simple. Relaxation exercises reverse the body's fight-or-flight mechanism. Relaxation exercises foster wellness and help to heal an oversensitive nervous system.

Let the wave of air travel from your belly first, and then exhale fully from your chest. Breathe slowly as you do this. You'll find this process quite relaxing. When you get the hang of it, teach your child to do it. You both will have fun lying on the floor together, seeing who can raise or lower the chest book or the belly book with the most control!

After your child understands how to trigger this relaxation response from breathing and eventually from the relaxation exercises, he can use this technique anywhere. He knows that the anxiety comes from his mind and his body. This technique harnesses his mind and his body to combat anxiety. On a blank tape, record the three exercises at the end of this chapter for your child. Then have him use the tape every day for a week. Notice whether your child records in his Journal that he is more relaxed.

## Exercise

Watch a playground full of kids. What do you see? Kids who are running, jumping, playing ball, swinging to the sky, and digging in the sandbox. Healthy kids are naturally active. Anxiety and depression can slow a child down, and this in turn can lead to the child being physically out of touch with his body. As a result, the child might not be able to sleep well at night. Research shows that physical exercise can actually reduce depression and can increase the amount of serotonin, a key neurotransmitter that is also increased by many antidepressants. There is a lot to like about exercise. How much exercise a child needs is variable. You may want to ask your child's PE teacher about the types of fitness evaluations that are conducted at his school. If your child participates in the

Presidential Physical Fitness Award program, you may want to see how he compares to national averages for his age. It is striking to note that an eight-year-old needs to run a mile in 8 minutes and 48 seconds to qualify for this award, and to be able to do 5 pull-ups and 40 sit-ups in a minute for each event! Clearly, kids can do amazing amounts of physical exercise. Yet many children today don't have the opportunity to go out and play after school that adults a generation ago enjoyed when they were kids.

After you establish how much exercise your child gets now and set some goals to improve his fitness, think about how to help him reach those goals. Many parents are also searching for ways to get more exercise. Perhaps you and your child could exercise together. Roller-blading, bike riding, running, walking, playing basketball or soccer—all offer fun, easily accessible ways for parents and kids to exercise together. Go to the local community pool as an after-school or weekend treat, walk to a local library or store, or race each other to the mailbox. If you start thinking of ways to help your child become more active, you'll find many that also work for your entire family. Jot down a few ideas for achieving greater physical fitness, and try them out with your kids.

## Parties and Play Dates

When your child's anxiety was really bad, the last thing on your mind was the importance of parties and play dates. Yet like other normal activities, these may need special attention as your child begins to recover. Ask your child to remember what his social life was like before his anxiety became so bad. If anxiety has been a problem for most of your child's life, you may not be able to start at this point. Begin by dreaming together with your child about how his social life might look if he weren't anxious.

A word of caution is in order here. Some kids, as they become less anxious, try too hard to become popular by making jokes that other kids don't find funny. This can be heartbreaking to a child who is trying out new social skills. It's important to remember that not every change in behavior will work out. That is part of social learning. Remind your child that the Dragon will try to make him see failure when every effort is not quickly rewarded. The Wizard way, though, is to see the many possible roles one can choose, ranging from being shy to being the class clown. If your child acts so silly that even kids don't think he is funny, what alternative new behaviors could he try that might work better? People see themselves in part by the reactions they get from their peers. What does your kid want the other children to see him as? Is this possible? Clearly, some changes are just not possible. Being the class hero or the "most popular" is not a reasonable goal—at least, not immediately. A child who isn't very athletic is unlikely to become the class jock overnight. But he could join a game on the playground or read the newspaper sports page at breakfast and talk knowledgeably to other kids about last night's game.

## Extracurricular Activities

One way to be sure your child gets more exercise is to encourage him to join a sports team. Extracurricular activities, in general, offer kids an opportunity to excel in a wide variety of arenas, not just in sports. Other activities are especially important for kids who have difficulty with school due to learning difficulties or low self-esteem from years spent living with anxiety and depression. All too often, anxious children and parents drop extracurricular activities while the primary arena of anxiety at school is explored. This is almost always a mistake. To many parents, it seems that a stressed, anxious student needs more time at home to do homework and to rest. We have found, however, that extracurricular activities give an

Exercise. Bah. Who needs it? I like it when your child focuses on things I make her worry about. How can she do my job well when she's busy playing softball? I say, let your child stay home and relax . . . or try to! A busy child is hard for me to influence. A child with nothing to do can really pay a lot of attention to me and my needs.

anxious child another setting in which to blossom, one that may play directly to his strengths.

Kurt, in Chapter 1, was not interested in sports. Gym was bad enough, as far as he was concerned. He was very happy limiting his exercise to running outside with his friends in the neighborhood or going on walks to the library with his mother. Kurt liked these noncompetitive activities, but he could see the advantage of extracurricular activities as a way to find more friends. Yet it would take him a while to trust the kids at school, because they had been cruel to him when he was depressed. Kurt looked around at various activities and found several that sounded interesting, including a one-week summer camp researching the Civil War with a college professor and a six-week pottery class for kids. Kurt's mom was astounded that these activities interested him, but she encouraged him nonetheless. She remembered that as a young child, before his anxiety and his learning disability became dominant forces in his life, Kurt was always interested in trying new things. His self-confidence and curiosity were traits that she had almost forgotten. These memories were rekindled with Kurt's new exploration of extracurricular activities.

## Breathing Script

(Read this script while your child listens and follows your instructions.)

Begin by lying with your back on the floor. Place your hand on your stomach. Now, breathe in slowly and fully; notice that you are lifting your hand with your stomach as air rushes deeply into your lower lungs. Think *air in* when you breathe in. As you breathe out, think *air out*. Breathe slowly, all the way in. Hold your breath. Pause. Now let the air all the way out.

Concentrate all of your attention on this simple act of breathing easily and fully. Gently close your eyes. *Air in, air out.* I will count backward from 10 to 1. As I count back, let yourself be more and more focused only on your breathing. Don't let any other thought come into your mind. If other thoughts try to come into your mind, gently stop them by saying, "Not now." Again, focus on the numbers and on your breathing.

- 10
- 9
- 8
- 7
- 6
- 5
- 4
- 3
- 2
- 1

Feel yourself floating quietly and gently. Now slowly open your eyes. Enjoy this peaceful feeling. Remember that focusing for a few seconds on your breathing can calm you anywhere, anytime.

## Relaxation Script

Think about relaxing your whole body for a few minutes. When you start this work, be sure that you are in a place where you can be quiet and still for a few minutes. Everyone needs to know how to relax. Imagine a baby sleeping. Nothing shows you better what it means to relax completely. Now think of the baby awake and looking at you. Think of the baby screaming because he is hungry. The same baby looks different asleep and relaxed, awake and alert, or screaming and hungry.

When you were a baby, your body relaxed even though you didn't know what your body was doing. Now that you are older, you can learn to relax so that your mind has a chance to take a break from thinking and worrying. Deep breathing gives your body and your mind a lovely little break.

Being relaxed means being quiet in your mind and your body. When you think about being relaxed, remember that sleeping baby—soft, warm, and quiet. Breathing quietly. Being peaceful.

Begin to relax by settling into a comfortable position. Find easy, comfortable places for your arms, your legs, and your head. Close your eyes gently.

Take three calming, deep breaths. Feel your stomach push out with each breath in. Feel your stomach sink in with each breath out. Think of the word *calm* each time you breathe out.

Now imagine that you can create a soft warm light that shines on your body. You will guide this light slowly over your body. As you shine the light on any part of your body, you feel the light warm your skin and make that part of your body warm, loose, and relaxed.

Imagine that the light is shining on your head. Feel your head grow warm and relaxed. Feel the skin around your eyes and mouth become warm and relaxed. Continue to breathe slowly and deeply.

Now shine the imaginary light on your neck and shoulders. Your shoulders become soft and relaxed as they warm from the spotlight in your imagination.

The light moves now, traveling down your arms to your hands. Feel your arms become heavy as they warm and relax. It may feel as if the warm light is traveling right out your fingertips, as your hands become warm and relaxed.

Take another deep breath and shine your magic light onto your stomach and back. Think about your back. Let it relax slowly. Feel your stomach relax and become calm. Let your legs relax as the warm light travels down your body. Let your knees relax and settle. Feel your lower legs relax and become warm and heavy. Feel the warm light flow through your feet and out your toes, as your feet become warm and relaxed.

Enjoy this feeling of being relaxed and calm. Let your body learn how this feels. Now that you know this feeling, it can be yours anytime you want. Simply recall the words *relaxed* and *calm*, and breathe easily, slowly, and deeply. Peace will return to you.

Now it is time to let the light go and to return to the world outside your body. You may feel like moving a little. Blink and open your eyes. Think about how good it feels to be awake and relaxed and calm. Smile to yourself. You did this for yourself. You deserve to feel this good. Take this peace with you as you rejoin your day.

When you are fearful, the blood flows out of your skin and into your muscles to prepare you for an urgent fight-or-flight response. For the same reason, the blood leaves your intestines when you face danger. When you shine an imaginary light on your body, your skin responds by taking in more blood, reversing the physiology of danger with the physiology of relaxation. Panic turns into relaxation, right in your skin. (McCarter. *Integrative Treatment of Anxiety Disorders*, 1996, 77–112)

## Travel Imagery Script

It is time to go to a special place in your imagination. This is the trip you have been looking forward to—this is your chance to go to your special place. It may be a real place where you have been that you remember. It may be a place you wish you could go but a place you haven't yet gone to. Or it could be a made-up place. This is your chance to choose where you go in your imagination. A place that exists only in your imagination. This is your own special place. This is your own imaginary trip.

Find a comfortable position and close your eyes. Imagine yourself climbing on board your personal shuttle. Transportation just the way you want it. Feel the seat cushion you in perfect comfort. You control the speed of your imaginary shuttle. You can go fast or slow; it's up to you. Think about where you are going. It is getting closer. Feel the wind on your face, and take a deep breath, as you feel totally safe.

You have arrived at your special place. This is where you have wanted to go. This is your own perfect place. Safe, warm, relaxing—being here is just what you want and need.

What do you see? What do you hear? Do you smell beautiful flowers? Can you feel warm sunshine on your arms and face? Take a few minutes to explore your special place. You feel welcome and safe here. Get to know this wonderful feeling. Let your mind roam, filled with happy thoughts. Let time pass.

Now it's time to leave your special place. Climb back into your own special shuttle. Before you leave, take a minute to feel the relaxation and peace you have experienced here. Know that this special place is all yours. You can return here as often as you like. The ride back on your imaginary shuttle seems to end much more quickly than the ride to your special place.

Begin to think about being here, now. This, also, is your special place. This is your unique life. You may find yourself shifting and moving as you return from your wonderful journey. Blink and open your eyes. Remember that wherever you are right now, this is your personal special place. Know it. Appreciate it. Explore it.

## Homework for Step 3

1. Have your child practice relaxation daily and record the practice in his Journal.
2. With your child, pick two goals for this week, using his anxiety goals as a guide, and plan two practice sessions.
3. Record or have your child record a description of his practice in his Journal.
4. With your child, rate how he is now, compared to how he was when you started working on Step 1. Worse? The same? Better? What has been the most helpful? What has been the least helpful?

### Action Steps

- Practice relaxation exercises with your child every day for a week. Spend ten minutes together doing these exercises or yoga, tai-chi, or meditation. You will both feel an increased sense of self-confidence as a result.
- Think about how your child is doing with his anxiety now, compared to when you started Step 1. Be sure to compliment him on his achievements.

CHAPTER 8

# Step 4

## *Rebecca's Story—School Anxiety and School Refusal*

Rebecca was fourteen when she had her first panic attack. She had always been shy, but suddenly, during a choir performance at the end of her ninth-grade year, Rebecca had to leave the stage because she felt sick and scared in front of all the people in the auditorium. Of course, the other kids in the chorus noticed her leave the stage. Rebecca felt totally humiliated by her weakness and fear. She hid in the bathroom until the end of the concert. She told her parents that she was sick when they drove her home. She looked sick—sick and very scared. That look frightened her parents. The next day they took her to the doctor, who said that Rebecca would be fine after a summer's rest. The doctor didn't understand how terrified she felt all the time. Rebecca was too embarrassed to tell the doctor about her fears. The next day, she didn't go to school. She just stayed in bed. Because only one week was left before the end of the school year, she had exams and papers to do. Rebecca didn't feel as if she could get out of bed. Her mom called the school to get the assignments for her to do during the summer.

When school was over for the year, Rebecca felt better. It was summer. She could read and work on her assignments and papers—which she actually liked to do—on her own. She went to

131

the pool every day and played with her dog. Rebecca was so happy that she almost forgot how scared she had been on stage with the chorus that night. But then, suddenly, it was the last week of August and time to buy school supplies. Rebecca was afraid of her fear coming back. It terrified her. On the first day of school, Rebecca stayed in bed. The next day she stayed in bed, too. The day after that, her mom took her to see a therapist, who taught her how to distract herself from her fears, and how to breathe deeply to reduce her level of anxiety. The therapist also told her about the Dragon that had scared her on stage with the chorus. Rebecca was amazed to learn that no matter how scared the anxiety Dragon made her feel, the Dragon couldn't hurt her. The therapist then said that she could find a Wizard in her own head to help tame the Dragon. Even though these ideas seemed simple to Rebecca, they made sense when she thought about how scared she felt. Right away, she started working on her Journal, writing about her Dragon and her Wizard. That day Rebecca also saw a psychiatrist, who gave her an antianxiety medicine to take when she got too scared.

Rebecca was glad the therapist and the psychiatrist understood what was wrong with her. She was also glad that they had things for her to do to get better. Rebecca really wanted to go back to school. She noticed that even at home, she still felt bad much of the time. After all, it wasn't summer any more, and there really was no place for a fourteen-year-old to be except in school. The pool was closed, and even going to the mall felt funny because no other kids were there.

The next day, Rebecca got on the school bus when it stopped in front of her house. She was going back to school four days late. She was worried about that and worried about becoming terrified, but she felt calmer with the medication. Rebecca remembered that one Wizard trick was to distract herself from thinking full time about her fear. When she sat by her friend on the bus and talked with her, she almost forgot about the Dragon. Rebecca now remembered how nice it felt to sit with her friends. She had predicted that her anxiety would be an 8 on the bus, but it only got to Level 4. She was sure that she could shift her thoughts away from a fear level of only 4.

The most amazing part of Rebecca's story was that after all that worry about going back to school, she didn't encounter any problems with her teachers or friends. No one knew how close she had come to missing weeks of school. Classes were still being shuffled around when Rebecca returned, so her showing up unexpectedly after missing four days was similar to what everyone did that first week. Rebecca's friends were busy with their own adjustments at the start of the year. They were glad she felt better, but they didn't know that anxiety had made Rebecca "sick" in the first place. Rebecca still had to work on her shyness and fear of singing in the chorus, but all of that was more manageable once she was back in school. She had a new sense of confidence because she understood what was happening to her. She had learned what anxiety was. She and her mother also had a lot of techniques to use when Rebecca felt anxious.

## Step 4: School Anxiety—Many Different Fears

Most, but not all, kids who suffer from anxiety worry a lot about school. If this particular form of anxiety doesn't apply to your child, it may seem strange that a safe, familiar place like school could be scary to some kids. Especially for kids who have just one fear, like needles or dogs, school is usually a safe place—no doctors or pets allowed! If your child doesn't worry about school, just skip over this chapter. Move right on to finding out the good things about anxiety in Chapter 12.

Most of you will read this chapter, because most kids worry a lot about school. The school day offers many opportunities for anxious students to worry. Your child has probably listed his school worries for you: teachers, your bus being in a different place and you can't find it, other kids, the order you are picked in gym to play soccer— all of these possible worries can poison the day for an anxious kid. The Dragon is ready to grab hold of these fears and make them grow very, very big.

I always make it hard for your child to start his homework practice sessions. I will keep bugging your child
until he does his practice. The only way to stop me
from bothering him is for him to just do the practice and get it
over with. I hope you and your child don't figure that out!

If your child has an acute problem with school right now, and
you have turned to this chapter before looking at any other part of
the book, you may find reading about Dragons, Wizards, and fear
levels a bit confusing. You will still get the main ideas in this chapter, but our techniques really work best if you also read the three
steps that go before this one. For now, it's important to understand
that we imagine anxious fear to be like a Dragon. The Dragon
seems terrifying and makes your child have powerful, unpleasant
physical feelings. The Dragon tells your child not to do the things
she fears, and this appears to reduce your child's fears for a time. In
the end, however, the limitations are too much for the child. This
is when school avoidance usually starts. School avoidance is a big
problem for kids, teachers, parents, and school systems. We have
included this specific step about school anxiety because kids need to
be in school. Anxiety can be a barrier to them staying there. This is
not to disagree with parents who have chosen to home school or
home tutor a child with severe anxiety. Remember, this book was
written for kids and parents in general. In our clinical experience,
school is the best place for a child to be. The environment may
need to be modified for special reasons, or children may need a special school to meet their needs, but school offers them a place to be
with other children and a rich environment for structured learning
that is tough to re-create at home without a tremendous amount of
work by the parent. If your child is home schooled and you are having trouble with his anxiety, you may need to adapt this chapter's
advice to your situation. For example, you may have to set up steps
for your child that include going to a friend's house to play, without
you being present, or going on a day field trip with another home-
schooling parent, to practice being separated from you.

We do not recommend home-schooling a child *because* of the child's anxiety (or, even worse, because of a parent's anxiety). For some children and families, there are good reasons to embark on home schooling, but the child having school anxiety is not an adequate reason. If you've read this book from the start, you know why we have reached this conclusion. Our recommendation has nothing to do with the merits of home schooling. Our general approach is that children need to face their anxiety and not avoid it. Avoidance just worsens the anxiety problem and compounds its handicapping effects. Our thinking about anxiety in adults is the same—avoidance is not the best solution. When talking to children about school anxiety, we often start with a clear statement that everyone has a job to do in life. For children, school is their job. It may take a while to get there, but everyone needs to have a clear goal from the outset. For a child with school phobia, that goal is to get back to school.

Some research shows that starting with hard tasks may help a child confront the fear of anxiety better than doing the step-wise goal progression, from easier to harder goals. Remember this as you send your child off to school. You can't go too fast, even if it is harder than doing one step at a time.

Remember that the key to taming the Dragon is to understand that it can't really do anything bad to your child. The Dragon wants your child to think that it can harm her, or it wants her to do certain things to protect the people she loves, but the Dragon can't really hurt her or anyone else. Your child's fear is the only food the imaginary Dragon in your child's mind can eat. The more your child fears her Dragon, the bigger and scarier it grows. The Dragon wants to make your child its prisoner, its pet. The Dragon wants your child to give up important parts of her life and feed and pay attention only to it.

Once your child understands these facts about the Dragon and has learned to calm herself down, she can turn and face the Dragon. As you worked through previous chapters, you helped your child understand the Dragon, set goals to practice facing the Dragon, and use her Wizard. You and your child have learned deep breathing and progressive relaxation. Your child is facing the things she fears. Her fear levels have probably started to go down.

To combat the Dragon, we ask you and your child to imagine a Wizard. This Wizard has magical tricks that help your child tame the Dragon. The six steps in Part Two of this book are designed to teach your child specific Wizard magic. The Wizard's techniques in this chapter are a bit different from those in the other steps, because school is a specific and complex situation. For this chapter, it's helpful to think about the problems that a kid has, based on the type of anxiety that he experiences. Remember, we haven't written this book only for children officially diagnosed with an anxiety disorder. Rather, our techniques may be used by parents of children who have mild problems that don't need therapist intervention, as well as by parents of kids who are being helped by professionals.

Now, with this review in mind, you will better understand the point we make about school anxiety. If your child has missed school due to anxiety, it's vital that you both understand that the more she stays away from school, the harder it is to go back. If she has missed one day of school, find something new to try from this book, so that she can go back to school tomorrow. If she has missed many days of school, try a new technique so that she can go back tomorrow, even if only for a few minutes. If she had a tough time staying in school today, look for something she can try tomorrow that will help her go to school.

Your child is better off if she goes back to school to face her fears! We don't ask out of meanness that your child face her fears, or because we don't take your child's anxiety seriously. We recommend that she go to school because we know that the more she avoids something she's afraid of, the harder it is to catch up on the work to get back to a full life. This is especially true with regard to school because your child can feel out of place in so many different ways when she has been out of school. She can feel out of step with her friends socially, as well as academically. She has to figure out how to explain her absence. If she tells the truth, that she missed school because she was scared, she risks being teased. This can be humiliating and can make returning to school even harder. If she just says she was sick, she risks feeling emotionally isolated from her friends, who will never know about her anxiety problem. This is a tough call. A mental health problem can still stigmatize both kids and adults.

She will also have to catch up on schoolwork. Even if she has been diligent about having homework sent to her and turns it all in when she goes back, it's tough to be in a class, readjusting, when the teacher could call on you at any minute.

Another problem about returning to school may be the change in sleep schedules. Most kids naturally stay up later and sleep later when they know that they don't have to be somewhere first thing in the morning. Returning to a school schedule can be especially tough for adolescents. This isn't a problem to take lightly. A child who has trouble with school and then feels tired in the morning will find a way to make his parent let him stay home in bed. Be sure that your child is getting plenty of physical, as well as mental, exercise during the day and insist that he is awake and active at a regular hour, even when he isn't in school due to a doctor's appointment or other reason. Set up a sleep window when your child is expected to be in bed and then record how closely he keeps to this schedule. It will take a few nights for your child to learn to go to sleep at the agreed-on time. Make a plan with him about what to do if he is awake in bed when it is time to sleep. May he read quietly with a flashlight or a table lamp for fifteen minutes? Or sing quietly to himself? We don't recommend watching TV or listening to music, nor do we recommend parents staying beside the child, as they did when the child was small. You want her to learn to go to sleep on her own so that she can re-create the experience of falling asleep in other places and in the middle of the night, should she awaken.

Many anxious children have a hard time letting go at night—getting into bed and falling asleep. They put off bedtime as long as someone else is up. Older anxious children will stay up even after others have gone to bed if they don't have to get up in the morning. Here is a general principle to follow with anxious children: Help your child keep a regular pattern of going to bed and getting up during the week so that no big shifts occur in his sleep schedule, whether he is in school or not. When his sleep time shifts, it disturbs the body's normal rhythms and further disrupts sleep. It's like having jet lag over and over again, but without the benefit and fun of travel. Shifting sleep patterns can increase anxiety in already anxious children. Setting a definite sleep schedule for your child can make a tremendous difference in how much anxiety your child experiences.

### Sleep Goal: Bed 9:30 P.M., Up 6:45 A.M.

| Date | Time actually in bed | Time actually up |
|------|---------------------|------------------|
|      |                     |                  |
|      |                     |                  |
|      |                     |                  |
|      |                     |                  |
|      |                     |                  |
|      |                     |                  |

On many mornings parents wonder whether they should send their anxious child to school. Typically, a child with school phobia will say that she feels sick. The parents feel torn about the situation. They should find out about the school's rules on illness. Most schools have clear guidelines, typically prohibiting kids with a serious communicable illness from attending. Also, if children have a fever or are throwing up, they should stay home and rest. If, however, children merely have a mild cold or complain of something minor, like a small cut or a sore stomach, they should go to school. Think about it as if you had this symptom and had an important meeting. You wouldn't cancel the meeting because of a mild problem. You would likely forget the minor problem altogether while in the meeting. If you were throwing up and had a fever with a stomach virus, though, you surely wouldn't go to that meeting! At a time when your child is calm, show her the school's list of illnesses that prohibit attendance. Help her understand that if she does get sick at school, help is available. Then, some morning when your child complains about a small symptom, remind her that the Dragon is probably playing a trick on her and the only way to escape from the Dragon's prison is by going to school that very day.

As you prepare to help your child get back to school after an absence, ask yourself whether she has any medication that can help her get through the tough moments. If she has never seen a doctor about her anxiety, it may be time to find one. Although we usually advise taking small steps when working on an anxiety problem, in this case it is so important for your child to get back to school that you should consider the option of medication. Even if she doesn't use it, you'll both feel better about her taking this scary first step of going back to school knowing that the medicine is an option. See Chapter 5 for advice on finding a doctor or a therapist. Medication can be really useful for calming anxiety. After she has settled into her school routine, she can work on the anxieties that kept her away.

Kids' fears about school usually fall into one of six types, with six matching diagnostic categories:

| Type of Symptom | Diagnostic Category |
| --- | --- |
| Fear of leaving home or leaving the safety of Mom or Dad. | Agoraphobia (Separation Anxiety) |
| Fear of having a panic attack. | Panic Disorder |

| Type of Symptom | Diagnostic Category |
|---|---|
| Fear of being the center of attention, like having to ask to go to the bathroom, fearing what other kids will say or do to embarrass you, or fear of not knowing the right answer in class. | Social Anxiety Disorder |
| Fear of closed doors or stairways, elevators, or heights. | Specific Phobia (Often Claustrophobia) |
| Fear of contamination, a need to perform ritual behaviors, or fear of harming others if things are not done just right. | Obsessive-Compulsive Disorder |
| Worry about the safety of parents or pets; worry about homework or keeping track of the schedule; multiple shifting worries | Generalized Anxiety Disorder |

Your child may not fall clearly and easily into any one category. Remember Rebecca at the beginning of this chapter? A parent might think that she fit the profile of either panic disorder or social anxiety disorder. Anxiety problems in general have a great deal of overlap between diagnoses. With children, it's often difficult even for a professional to make a clear distinction between types of anxiety problems. Kids seem to have a blending of different problems, almost as if the Dragon were trying to find out which problem would bother your child the most. For now, simply think about which anxiety profile fits her best, and then refer to that section for specific techniques.

## Fear of Leaving Home—Agoraphobia

Joseph was a nine-year-old chatterbox. He had lots of friends and played on several sports teams outside of school. No one who saw this big, friendly kid could believe that he hated to be away from his home or his mom. Most of the time, this worked out fine because Joseph and his mom didn't have to be apart. His mom volunteered at school. She liked to knit and talk to the other parents while she watched his soccer practice. She assumed that Joseph would grow out of his intense attachment to her, but he didn't. In the third grade it began to get worse, instead of better. He wanted his mother to be at the beginning of the carpool line every day—not just one of the first cars, but the very first car in line. This meant that Joseph's mom had to arrive half an hour before school was over to wait in the car, knitting. Then Joseph became upset because his brother's soccer practice was scheduled at the same time as his. This meant that his mother had to drop him off and drive his brother to a different location. Joseph was so scared by the idea of her leaving him alone at the field that he wouldn't go to soccer one day. He cried inconsolably, all the way to his brother's practice. His mother was alarmed. The idea of Joseph's feeling of being alone, despite the presence of a team full of friends, a coach, and several mothers, made her realize that she was dealing with an irrational anxiety. The situation seemed complicated because only she saw this side of Joseph.

Joseph's mom found a book about people with anxiety. Gradually, she explained some of the book's ideas to Joseph. He was glad that she didn't blame him for missing soccer and for making her volunteer in the library in order to stay at school with him. It helped both of them tremendously to understand that the Dragon made him anxious about his mom because the Dragon knew that Joseph loved his mom so much. That made sense. Joseph realized that he would need help from the Wizard to beat this thing. Besides, Joseph had a really important goal: He wanted to stop being scared to leave his mom so that he could go to a friend's birthday slumber party next month.

A little phrase in this book helped Joseph a lot. It was "My mom loves me even if she is not here." It seemed simple, but using the Wizard's magic by saying this phrase when he was scared really helped. He was especially scared to practice letting his mom not be first in the carpool line, but he knew that she had to get her own life back. She could no longer spend so much time waiting for him. He tried a new Wizard magic trick. In the afternoon, when he felt scared looking out his classroom window and saw that his mom wasn't in the line of cars, he imagined a favorite song playing in his head. This trick was especially good because the kids had to sit quietly while the carpools were called. Joseph found that he almost never got all the way through the song in his head before his carpool was called. Instead of dreading the wait, he began to hope she would arrive later, because he enjoyed this exercise so much.

Joseph made it to the slumber party at his friend's house. He used his Wizard tricks, saying, "My mom loves me even though she is not here," and singing a song in his head. The party was fun. Joseph felt even closer to his mom since they had both worked so hard to overcome this tough anxiety problem.

## Fear of Having a Panic Attack: Panic Disorder

At the beginning of this chapter, fourteen-year-old Rebecca had a panic attack on stage during a chorus performance. She was so terrified by the baffling, strong feelings that she just wanted to stay home in bed. She felt as if something was really wrong with her. She responded by acting sick. Her reaction is understandable. Her parents acted reasonably, too, given that their daughter was clearly upset and felt so sick. Sometimes people will have an isolated panic attack like this, and it never happens again. They will find it upsetting but won't associate it with any particular experience or place. Rebecca did associate her panic attack with a place—school. That's why she could go through the whole summer without a panic attack and then feel panic again when the fall semester drew closer.

Why was Rebecca so afraid to have a panic attack at school? Why didn't she have similar fears of a panic attack at home or somewhere else? Remember, when children have panic attacks, they think that they are desperately ill, could pass out, or could even die right at that moment. Some children feel more vulnerable, and less cared for, at school. They may feel safer at home, especially if a trusted parent is with them. After you understand how a panic attack works, you can see why children react as they do.

Panic attacks are very frightening if you don't know anything about the Dragon and the Wizard. Knowing that the Dragon couldn't harm her with panic symptoms helped Rebecca, but that knowledge didn't take away the anticipatory anxiety that made it more likely that she would have another panic attack. Being able to use medication was a Wizard trick that helped her a lot. Not only did this mean that she could stop a panic attack if necessary, having medication available also showed Rebecca that something physical was happening in her body during the panic attack. She had been afraid that she was going crazy. Knowing that the panic symptoms were caused by a real condition in her brain helped her understand that she could learn to manage this problem, just as she managed any other physical problem.

## Fear of Attention: Social Phobia

Some kids are shy. Others are quiet. Shy and quiet personality traits can be useful and can endear a kid to the adults around her. On the other hand, a shy, quiet child may be so terrified of being the focus of attention that she fears being called on in class. In this case, the child is upset and stays quiet to avoid attracting any attention at all. This can be a major problem, as the child avoids situations where she has to speak up. Jenny was a shy eleven-year-old who had few friends at school. She was terrified of getting into trouble, which seemed unlikely to happen because she carefully followed every rule her teacher laid out. She was also terrified of her classmates teasing her. This was harder to avoid because her withdrawn nature made her an easy target. Jenny was making it through school academically, although the teacher conferences always involved her teacher asking her parents to encourage her to speak up in class, since she clearly knew most of the answers. The teachers knew this because Jenny got such good grades.

One day Jenny developed a bladder infection. She had been limiting how much she drank during the day so that she wouldn't have to raise her hand in class to ask to go to the restroom. Her pediatrician identified the bladder infection as a problem that would likely reoccur unless she received help for her shyness, so the family was referred to a child psychiatrist. Everyone in the family was shocked by this. Jenny's parents had accepted her quiet personality, yet they had to recognize that their daughter had developed a health problem as an indirect result of her shyness.

The psychiatrist educated the family about the Dragon and gave Jenny specific Wizard tricks to try. Since the Dragon was trying to limit how much attention Jenny got in school, the doctor urged her to think about the attention of her teacher and her classmates as positive, negative, or neutral. Most interaction with others falls into the last category, the psychiatrist explained. The Dragon, of course, wanted Jenny to see all interactions as negative. Jenny set up a chart in her Journal to keep track of her interactions at school. She was surprised to find that most were neutral, as the psychiatrist had predicted.

High levels of physical activity in school-aged children help to improve developing self-esteem and belief in one's own ability to handle situations and successfully follow through on goals. (Strauss, et al. *Archives of Pediatric and Adolescent Medicine*, vol. 155, no. 8 [August 2001]: 897–902)

At times, negative comments are made, even about a good girl like Jenny. Learning how to cope with negative interactions without falling apart is an important part of childhood. Jenny used some of the negative comments she recorded in her Journal in order to come up with sitcom responses. This Wizard trick let her pretend that she was someone else who was able to answer a hard question. She learned that she didn't have to use all the answers that her Wizard-transformed alter ego came up with. Still, it was a relief to realize that she actually could think of good responses to negative comments, even if it took her days! Previously, she had avoided thinking about the bad things people said, but now, after recording the negative statements, she found very few to work with. Eventually, patterns of communication appeared. Jenny was able to use her stockpile of new or clever responses when people made negative comments. One boy in her class teased her by staring at her. She used to blush, drop things, and be unable to concentrate, until the boy laughed at his ability to upset her without saying a single word. Jenny learned to stare right back, without blinking. The boy was unable to hold her gaze! He turned away in defeat. What a sense of accomplishment that was for Jenny!

It's interesting how we came up with the Wizard trick of pretending to be someone else, for kids who have social phobia. Remember Rebecca's story, about a girl whose panic attacks began in a public place, while she sang in a choir production? Rebecca had a panic disorder, not social phobia. She feared school because that's where her first panic attack happened. Her core fear was that she would again have that panicky feeling. Kids with social anxiety are often quite good at performing, either in a play or another group setting, where they act in a role someone else has given them. One kid said that he felt good performing, because all he had to do was memorize someone else's lines. He didn't have to figure out what to say himself on stage. Not all socially anxious kids will find this to be true, but you may be surprised at how secure your socially anxious child feels in having lines or a chorus part to memorize.

---

Does your child long to be back in school so that she can perform in the spring musical or be part of the chess team? Find a flyer from school or a school logo to put in her Journal, as a reminder of the good things she will experience when she goes back.

---

Jenny also had to practice raising her hand in class to go to the restroom. She did this to get over her fear, because the pediatrician told her to drink more liquids and to go to the restroom more often. This was tough at first. Jenny would wait all during class and get up her courage at the very end. Waiting solved one problem, though; the teacher and the other kids weren't focused on Jenny because the class changed at that point. Yet waiting until the end of class meant that the entire time Jenny worried about raising her hand and couldn't focus on the lesson. The Dragon had found power over Jenny by making her dread the moment she raised her hand. The more she put that moment off, the more time the Dragon had to bother her. Jenny found that it was far better to raise her hand at the beginning of class and get it over with. Then she could concentrate during the rest of the class without the Dragon bothering her.

Jenny continued to be a shy girl, but now she was a confident shy girl who could stand up for herself and answer questions in class. She didn't get any more bladder infections, and she felt better about herself overall after facing her fears.

## Fear of Closed Doors: Specific Phobia

Seven-year-old Tanya's family went to the beach for spring vacation. They all had a great time, but on the last day of vacation Tanya thought that she was locked in the bathroom, alone. She was terrified. Only after another woman went into the ladies room did her mother and father hear about Tanya's upsetting ordeal. She had mistaken a locked broom closet for the exit and had panicked to find the door locked. No matter how hard she tried, she couldn't open that door to get to her parents.

The family was about to drive out of town when this happened. They tried to quiet Tanya's crying by saying that she had never been in any danger. On the drive home, Tanya wouldn't use the restrooms at the rest stop. She made her father pull the car over in a secluded area so that she could empty her bladder behind a tree. No danger of being trapped there! Tanya's parents were at a loss. They didn't know how to cope with this. They hoped that everything would go back to normal the next day when Tanya returned to school.

Instead, things got worse. Tanya noticed that not only were the school restrooms behind closed doors, but that her teacher kept the classroom door closed. Tanya cried so much that her teacher opened the door a crack. Tanya asked her to prop it open with a book so that it wouldn't blow closed by accident. The next day at school the teacher propped the classroom door open, but then Tanya had to use the restroom and was afraid that its door would close. She asked a friend to hold the restroom door open while she used the toilet, but she felt terrible about not having privacy. Later, when her class had PE, Tanya discovered, while walking to the gym, that the closed doors at the top and the bottom of the stairway made that stairway another place where she could be stuck. Instead of entering the enclosed stairwell, Tanya went to the nurse and asked to go home.

Adolescents with a high level of dental phobia are more likely than their normal peers to have other psychological diagnoses, such as conduct disorder, agoraphobia, social phobia, simple phobia, or alcohol dependence. Of the group with the highest levels of dental phobia, those who had an additional diagnosis were more likely to have had a longer history of dental anxiety. (Locker, et al. *Community Dental and Oral Epidemiology*, vol. 29, no. 6 [December 2001]: 456–463)

Tanya's mother and father took her to a child psychiatrist right away. They knew what had upset their little girl and wanted her to feel better quickly. The psychiatrist prescribed an antianxiety medication to use for a few days to help Tanya worry less and sleep better. He explained to Tanya and her parents how important it was for her to go to school. With their permission, he called Tanya's teacher, giving his approval for the way that she kept the door open, but without the book doorstop, for the next week. This allowed Tanya some extra time to practice going to the restroom with the door closed and walking up the stairway to PE. Tanya liked this compromise. She liked knowing that the Dragon couldn't hurt her. She found that the memory of what happened in the restroom at the beach was beginning to fade. She had to do more work to get back to her usual self, but she was on the road to recovery.

The Wizard magic for specific phobias generally involves a child taking small steps to get to the ultimate goal. Keeping a clear goal in mind and letting the child choose the next steps to try will work wonders, because your child can master her anxieties through practice.

## Fear of Contamination: Obsessive-Compulsive Disorder

Chapter 7, Step 3, begins with William, a boy with obsessive-compulsive disorder (OCD). William's story is useful because it reflects not only OCD but also Tourette's syndrome. Tourette's syndrome includes a pattern of involuntary noises and tics. Tics are rapid, meaningless movements such as eye blinking and neck jerking. Other tic disorders not accompanied by noises are also sometimes associated with OCD in kids. The research is still evolving about the relationship of OCD and Tourette's syndrome or tic disorder. Although there is clearly overlap, with groups of kids with OCD having a higher than expected incidence of tics, the genetic linkage between the two conditions is unclear. Behavioral therapy is helpful with tics, however. This involves practice in resisting the motion or making the noise, even though the impulse is present. Kids generally do well with this practice, because they don't want people to see them tapping their desks or jerking their shoulders. When kids first begin therapy to resist the tic movements, they do well to sit on their hands or hold their shoulders in such a way that they can't give in to the tic. This reprograms the child's brain so that she doesn't have to carry out the movement. As with other types of behavioral therapy, the beginning—when the child first must resist the movement—is intensely anxiety-provoking. Over time, the Wizard will help your child win if she works at it. Tics and Tourette's syndrome vary in their severity. If your child has mild problems, she can start with the behavior modification practices listed here. If she has a severe problem with tics, she should see a psychiatrist about medication. Medication for tics and Tourette's syndrome is different from that for OCD, which is one clue that researchers are investigating to determine whether these are in fact two different disorders that frequently co-occur or whether they are closely related.

> Selective mutism is classified as an anxiety-linked problem, but it also appears to have a strong neuro-logical component. There may be family communication styles that are learned in selective mutism, as well. All of this suggests that clear evaluations of neurological, psychological, and familial components in the child's life need to be assessed to maximize treatment results. (Kristensen. *European Child and Adolescent Psychiatry*, vol. 11, no. 2 [April 2002]: 71–78)

Relaxation helped William with some of his anxiety about the unpredictable Tourette's noises, which in turn reduced the amount of time he spent whistling. Relaxation also helped him to breathe slowly, which kept him from being able to whistle. Before he narrowed his problem down to that involuntary whistle, William spent a lot of time away from school. His refusal to go to school was different from that of other children we described in this chapter. Obsessive-compulsive disorder typically makes people think that something bad will happen to them or to someone else if they don't do things just right. William felt that with his hands covered in germs from the basketball, if he touched anything else, he might harm a friend or someone in his family. He wasn't that scared for himself; after all, he had already been contaminated. He was terrified for others whom he might harm. Any hand washing he did was useless, because his hands would then touch his contaminated clothing. Even after he took off his "dirty" clothes, showered, and put on clean clothes, his "dirty" self had walked through the hall to the restroom, so he immediately became dirty again when he left the restroom. If your child has problems like William's, you know how perplexing they can seem to another person. The concept of clean and dirty is so complicated, it's almost magical. What looks dirty, like a dirty plate on the kitchen table, may actually be clean to the person with OCD. If it is *the* clean plate and *the* clean part of the table, the dried food is irrelevant. Contamination seems to travel by thoughts and not by germs. Contamination is not like any dirt or germs you have ever known. Remember, these scary, upsetting thoughts are stuck in your child's mind, repeating over and over again. It's impossible to answer his questions about harm in any rational way, when they start from such an irrational source as the anxiety Dragon. The Wizard tricks show you that these irrational thoughts are false alarms. Your child's mind gets stuck on an OCD thought, and he feels an emotional response, with physical symptoms like a fast pulse rate and sweating.

> Cognitive-behavioral therapy alone, without any medication, was found to be statistically beneficial after twelve weeks of treatment in children who had obsessive-compulsive disorder. (Benazon et al. *Behavioral Research Therapy*, vol. 40, no. 5 [May 2002]: 529–539)

The stuck idea, paired with the intensity of the emotion and the physical symptoms, all make him think that this is a dreadful problem. The reality is that like a fire drill at school, it's a false alarm. There is actually no reason for your child to listen to the alarm of danger or respond to it. The Wizard trick is to help your child understand that even though it feels like a serious problem, it's a false alarm. He doesn't have to pay attention to it. This practice is called exposure and response prevention. Your child exposes himself to what he is afraid of and prevents himself from responding to his anxiety (the obsessions) the way the Dragon says he must (with compulsions and tics).

Combine this new way of thinking with having your child practice staying in difficult situations, over and over again, and he will tame the Dragon, even if his OCD was quite severe to begin with. The Dragon simply cannot continue when your child and the Wizard say that this is a false alarm and your child repeatedly practices difficult situations until these are no longer upsetting. The Dragon may attempt to change what your child obsesses about—for example, instead of germs in the cafeteria, it might be a fear of getting AIDS from the communion wine. Simply recognize that wherever the Dragon turns up, the intensity of the emotion and the fact that other people don't have the alarm are the giveaways that this is actually OCD, not a reasonable danger to take precautions against. Help your child return to the simple idea that the worry is a false alarm, and practice Wizard magic every day with him.

## Worry: Generalized Anxiety Disorder (GAD)

Ryan didn't worry when he was young. At thirteen, he was a busy, happy kid who helped around the house and got good grades in school by working hard. Then his father moved out, and his parents got divorced. Suddenly, he began to worry about everything. At night he worried about someone breaking into the house. That kept him awake for hours. In the morning it was tough to get up, so he worried about being late to school. He actually missed the bus several times because he got up so late that there was no way to catch it on time. Ryan worried in each class that he would have so much homework to complete, he wouldn't get to sleep on time. He worried after school that he'd miss the bus home. He had a hard time concentrating on anything, except his worries. School became just one more place to worry. This made him crabby and difficult for his mom to be around.

Because Ryan lived with his mom, his dad blamed her for Ryan's new worries. His mother felt guilty. Neither of them knew how to help Ryan except by letting him stay home from school to catch up on his sleep. This helped in one way, because he was less tired, but then he worried more than ever about keeping up with his class.

Ryan's mom went to a therapist for help. She didn't know if Ryan needed help, but she knew that *she* did.

> I'm good at making you think that something is seriously wrong. Just keep listening to me and focusing on those bad feelings I give you. That's what I want you to do. Keep feeding me with your child's fears. I'm happy if I scare you, too—that way, both of you are feeding me!

This situation was bad for the whole family. Ryan wasn't unreasonable in his response to the painful breakup of his parents' marriage. He had lost the security he had known. Sometimes anxiety will start like this, with a clear triggering event and a definite reason for the worry. Ryan's parents were divorcing. They would not get back together. Ryan needed a way to heal and move on, even in the face of this devastating change in his life. Giving in to the Dragon wouldn't solve anything. The "What if" questions, which are the bedrock of all anxious worries, had opened up for Ryan. He didn't have panic attacks and didn't worry about having them. Instead, he worried more or less all the time about what might happen. Even though his parents told him that they loved him and would always care for him, this sudden change in his living situation was proof that anything could happen. Ryan now knew that nothing was secure.

On a cognitive level, Wizard magic for GAD works best when the child who is worrying excessively and inappropriately can command himself, "Stop!" This strong statement stops the cascade of worries that otherwise completely distracts the child from focusing on and enjoying life in the here and now. Ryan found that when his mom suggested that he tell the Dragon to stop its shenanigans, he did feel better. Nevertheless, the problems in Ryan's life remained. Life wasn't as fun or secure as it had been, but at least he could interrupt the incessant chant of worries in his head. Ryan realized that no matter how bad the situation was with his parents' divorce, giving in to the Dragon made him even more unhappy.

Ryan then tried a Wizard trick that comes naturally to kids who worry a lot, whether they have a real, new problem in their lives or an out-of-proportion worry that the Dragon has created. Ryan drew a line down the center of a page in his Journal. Then he wrote all of his worries in one long list, down the lefthand side of the page. Some of these were worries that he could do nothing about; others, he could do something about. Yet others were things that had happened or were just worried Dragon thoughts about what *might* happen. He didn't stop to figure out which was which; he just wrote them all down.

When he was done, he sorted the worries into four categories: things to talk to his mom about; things to talk to his dad about; things to work on alone; and things to change his attitude about. For example, he needed to check out his worry about being orphaned with his mom and his dad. They both comforted him about the sadness of the situation and let him know that other people, like his grandparents, aunts, and friends, would care for him if anything happened to either of his parents. Ryan felt better about this. Just knowing that he would be taken care of, if something even worse happened, made him less worried about the future.

Most of Ryan's worries, he could see now, were things that he had to deal with using skills from Step 2 (cognitive restructuring). Ryan didn't think about it in those terms. He just remembered the Wizard step of transforming "What if" thoughts into "What is" facts, to get back to what's happening right now. He recognized that even though he couldn't control his family, he did have a lot of good choices in his life.

Ryan cheerfully went back to school. He calculated that his grades would be a little lower for now, but that was all right because he had learned a lot of other things while away from school. He learned that there are some bad things he couldn't fix, but that he could work on a lot of other things successfully.

## Posttraumatic Stress Disorder (PTSD)

Morgan was fifteen when her mother announced her plan to remarry. Morgan had never known her father; her parents had divorced when she was only one year old. Her father had never been in contact with her after that. Morgan didn't particularly like the man her mother planned to marry, but she was glad to see her mother so happy. Morgan's mom and new stepfather went to Las Vegas for a week, where they got married and spent their honeymoon. Morgan stayed with her best friend. She was so busy with school and field hockey practice that she didn't think much about how life would be when her mother and her stepfather returned.

When they did return, the whole family moved back to the apartment where Morgan and her mother had lived for many years. Then Morgan's stepfather began to sexually abuse her. Nothing in Morgan's life had prepared her for this horror, the secret-keeping and the shame of the experience. The final discovery by her mother was a big relief. Morgan's mother called the police and the stepfather was arrested. He never lived in the apartment again. Morgan's mother started divorce proceedings immediately. However, Morgan was terribly upset by what had happened. She slept poorly and startled easily. She hated being at home, so she spent as much time as possible with her friends. Since her friends didn't know what had happened, it was possible for Morgan to pretend that everything was fine while she was at school or socializing. Yet Morgan couldn't sleep and seldom stayed home, in an attempt to avoid her almost constant panic. All of this caused her to feel more upset. Her bad feelings began to affect her grades and her ability to play on the field-hockey team.

Her mother brought her to see a psychiatrist after Morgan stayed out one entire night. She had slept outside a friend's house, desperate to get some rest in a place that felt safe. Her home no longer did. Morgan and her mother were both in tears during the therapy session. Nothing could change the horrible fact of what had happened to Morgan. Her mother felt guilty for not having kept her daughter safe. Even though the stepfather was in jail and

Morgan had visited a gynecologist and was healthy, the emotional pain continued to devastate both of them.

The psychiatrist reminded Morgan and her mom that what had happened was terrible, but it was over. The Dragon was making Morgan relive her bad experience over and over again, because the Dragon knew that the memory of the abuse frightened her more than anything. Morgan didn't want to attend a group for sexual abuse survivors because she was afraid to hear other people's stories. The psychiatrist urged her to think about working with her mother, and on her own, to face the horror of her own story, instead of constantly fighting against it. The Dragon would only draw more power from her avoidant thoughts. The psychiatrist urged Morgan to write about the experience in short, five-minute blocks of time while at home, with her mother in the same room but not watching what Morgan wrote. The writing was Morgan's way of facing the Dragon. The psychiatrist said that her anxiety would go up when she spent time in the room where the abuse had happened and when she wrote about the abuse. He also told her that she could keep reminding herself that nothing was happening to her at that moment. The problem was over; she was safe now. At the end of her five minutes of writing, Morgan had a choice. She could keep what she had written, or she could, with her mother's help, burn each page as she wrote it. Knowing that the stepfather was in jail, the psychiatrist urged Morgan to begin sleeping in her own room again. He reminded her that the Dragon would continue to torment her until she faced those memories in her room and placed them firmly in the past. She hadn't wanted the abuse to happen. She was furious that it had. Yet she also had choices now that would let her move on with her life. Those choices included staying in school and participating in field hockey. To do those things, she would need sleep. Those were her first priorities.

Morgan practiced these techniques, finding them helpful. Her mother also decided to enter therapy, to deal with the guilt she felt about the terrible situation she had put her daughter in. The two of them spent quite a bit of time together, working on being a mother and daughter again, after the devastating trauma that had occurred.

Journals that are kept on a computer need illustrations, too. Try using a kid's art program to let your child add some personal art. Or scan in a picture that she has drawn with crayons. Personal Journals hold a lot of important information. They can be fun and creative, too.

They faced that work as a team. Even when they were angry with each other, as mothers and daughters normally are at certain times during the teen years, they remained truthful to and respectful of each other. They had learned that cruelty could come right into their own home. They didn't need to have cruelty between them. They loved each other far too much to let that happen. That would be a further victory for the cruelty of the stepfather and another prison of isolation imposed by the Dragon. Morgan and her mother didn't let that second mental victimization happen to them.

Ultimately, Morgan and her mother moved into a new apartment in the same school district. Their new home had no sad stories haunting the rooms where they lived. By the time they left the old apartment, Morgan could sleep in her room without difficulty. She was glad to move with her mother, although she knew that it was important not to run away from the old place before she faced the Dragon on her own terms. She saw that it really was just a room, not the House of Horrors that the Dragon made her think it was.

> "You are a girl Dragon, aren't you?!"
> —THE DONKEY, IN THE MOVIE *SHREK*.

## Homework for Step 4

1. Have your child think about any trouble that she has with school. Have her describe in her Journal what is wrong, and what she would think about this if she had no anxiety problem.

2. Have your child set a specific goal for this week in school. It may be to catch the bus on time every day, to talk to one new person each day, or to raise her hand in class one time.

3. As always, have her set two new goals for practice sessions this week. Continue to have your child record her anxiety levels in the Journal.

4. Have your child add a column to her practice Journal, to record how satisfied she is with her progress at each practice session. She can rate her feelings about her practice session as unsatisfied, satisfied, or very satisfied.

### *Action Steps*

- Get help from a psychiatrist or a pediatrician if you think that medication, even for a few days, would help your anxious child return to school.

- Remember that your child's practice in difficult situations, even when it's hard, leads to lower anxiety levels in the long run.

- Keep in mind all of the good things about your child being in school.

- Modify your child's routine or schedule if she needs to get back to school quickly, and then deal with the other problems later.

CHAPTER 9

# Step 5

## *Rebecca's Story One Year Later: Set Goals for the Future, Including a Plan If the Anxiety Problem Comes Back*

Rebecca returned to school four days late from summer vacation and continued in tenth grade with no more problems from the Dragon. Sometimes she used the ideas she had learned, but mostly, she didn't need the Wizard. She had a great fall. She made some new friends, played on a recreational volleyball team, and got almost all As on her report card. Her memory of her fight with the anxiety Dragon faded. For winter break Rebecca went on a special trip to the Caribbean with her parents to sail, something her family had wanted to do for years. They had a great time, relaxing, reading, and learning more about sailing, a hobby they passionately shared.

Spring semester at school started with no problems. By that time Rebecca had almost completely forgotten about the missed days of school the previous fall. She took difficult classes and spent most of her time outside of school studying. During spring break, she stayed at home, happily working on a complicated science experiment. Then, suddenly, it was time for Rebecca to start rehearsing for the spring choir concert. This was the one-year anniversary of the event when she had experienced her first panic attack.

Without warning, Rebecca began to have trouble falling asleep at night. She felt shy around her friends. She talked less to every-one. People didn't call her or invite her over to their houses as much, partly because she was now so quiet. Rebecca got very scared again. It all seemed like a bad dream—the anxiety Dragon was back. She could hardly remember all the good moments she had recently experienced. This time, though, Rebecca knew what to do. She told her parents about the Dragon's return. She opened her Journal to remember how to use the Wizard's help.

Her parents were upset that the anxiety was back, but they were glad to learn why Rebecca had suddenly become so quiet. They reminded her that she had beaten the Dragon before. There was a lot she could do to help herself. First of all, her dad reminded her that she hadn't played a sport in the spring, because she had been so busy with classes. The two of them started going for an evening bike ride, a run, or a walk every day. Rebecca's mom reminded her that she could take medication to reduce the anxiety and then called the psychiatrist's office to get a refill so that Rebecca wouldn't worry about running out of pills. Rebecca also remembered that she had liked doing relaxation exercises so she had her best friend record a new tape of her favorite exercise. Then she practiced lis-tening to the tape every night before bed. Rebecca's sleep improved immediately. Within three days Rebecca felt back to normal, with no anxiety. She had found her Wizard again. All of her old tech-niques worked against the Dragon. She had missed only half a day of school, to go to her psychiatrist's office for a medication appoint-ment. She felt full of pride that she had stopped the Dragon from

> All at once there was a scraping noise and the egg split open. The baby Dragon flopped onto the table. It wasn't exactly pretty; Harry thought it looked like a crumpled, black umbrella. Its spiny wings were huge compared to its skinny jet body; it had a long snout with wide nostrils, the stubs of horns and bulging, orange eyes.
>
> —J. K. ROWLING. *HARRY POTTER AND THE SORCERER'S STONE*
> (NEW YORK: SCHOLASTIC TRADE, 1997)

robbing her of her time at school the way it had the year before. At
her choir concert, Rebecca smiled as she sang. She felt no anxiety.
And at the end of the concert, her parents took her out for a surprise dinner at her favorite restaurant to celebrate the victory they
had won together.

## Step 5: Plan for the Future

In Step 4 you read about Rebecca and how she missed the end of
ninth grade and the first four days of tenth grade because she was
scared of school and of the panicky feelings the Dragon caused.
Here, you see that Rebecca's story had an important sequel. At the
end of tenth grade, she had another choir concert. As you will
recall, a situation can be a trigger for anxiety to come back. An
event where someone experienced anxiety before can be another
trigger. With Rebecca, you'll notice that no one thing led to her
anxiety returning. She hadn't done as much exercise, which may
have contributed to her problem with falling sleep. Once she was
tired, it was easier for the Dragon to scare her with the panicky
feelings she felt at choir rehearsal. Changes in your child's life can
make her get off track in keeping the Dragon away. A move, a new
school year, or even a change in the type of lunch that is available
can all be triggers for a child's anxiety to return. Situations or even,
as in Rebecca's example, times of the year can be triggers causing
the return of anxiety.

 I may come back in the same form or in a different
form. I can come back soon. But I can also wait a
long, long time to come back. I'm tricky.

Quickly reaching out for help was a crucial step for Rebecca. She
used help from her parents and saved a lot of time by finding her
Journal, so that she could immediately re-use the Wizard tricks that
helped her in the past.

Anxiety can come back even if it has been gone a long time. When it does come back, the Dragon may make your child feel that things will never get any better, that the anxiety problem was always this bad. The Journal offers her immediate help, written in her own words. Now, while you're using these techniques on your child's anxiety problem, make a plan for what you'll do if the Dragon finds your child again.

> In your child's Journal, keep track of books, web sites, mental health professionals, and other people, along with names and phone numbers, that have helped you and your child overcome the Dragon. If you need these resources again, they will all be together in one spot.

This story shows why it's especially important for your child to write down details of her recovery from anxiety. After her initial success, Rebecca forgot about the Dragon altogether. If she hadn't had her Journal and been able to tell her parents what was wrong, she would have had to backtrack before she could work on getting better. Another thing Rebecca did right was to figure out early on that the Dragon was back. This was quite scary for Rebecca. She didn't want the Dragon to be back. She spent an entire day pretending to herself that she was just coming down with a cold, and that the Dragon wasn't really back in her life.

> If your child is already involved in extracurricular activities that bring him joy, take a picture of him being active and happy. Tape the photo in his Journal. Or make a copy of a picture showing a fun activity that your child used to do and put it in the Journal, as a future goal.

Remind your child not to run from the Dragon! That's how it grows! When Rebecca told herself and her parents that the Dragon was back, then turned and faced the Dragon, she got rid of it in just three days. If she had waited longer and if the Dragon had become more of a problem, it might have taken a lot longer to beat it again. Respect what the Dragon can do, but don't fear it. Have your child tell the Dragon that whenever it bothers her, she is ready to tame it again.

Anxiety may take different forms than you'd expect. Children with asthma who suffered from breathlessness that couldn't be explained by lung-function testing were found to be triggered into thinking that they were breathless when, in fact, equipment that caused their skin to itch was being used. This sensation of itching was then translated by some children into a sensation of breathlessness. The use of lung-function testing is helpful in this type of situation to verify symptoms that may be anxiety-caused. (Rietveld et al. *Psychological Medicine*, vol. 29, no. 1 [January 1999]: 121–126)

## Finding the Good in Anxiety

Many parents see the good that indirectly comes from their child having an anxiety problem. After their initial surprise at the idea, most kids are also able to see that there are many good aspects to their anxiety. This doesn't mean that we think it's great to have an anxiety problem—rather, that something good can accompany a tough or painful part of life. This goal of finding the good in anxiety can be like a spiritual quest. If your family is religious, you may want to think about the spiritual implications of discovering good in something that seems bad on the surface.

Use a video camera, a digital camera, or a tape player to record your child performing or reading his tale of victory over the Dragon.

Even if the only benefit you can find is that the anxiety problem has allowed you to know your child better, that is a precious thing. It's something to celebrate. If you're having trouble with this assignment, you may want to ask a friend for help with it. Or try asking your anxious child. He just might surprise you with his answers.

> Allow yourself and encourage your child to dream about big goals. The Dragon has prevented him from hoping. Only by having dreams can he make good choices about working hard at school and recognize the importance of extracurricular activities. Help him think of the steps he can do right now that would move him toward his goals.

## Homework for Step 5

1. Review your child's next goals with him. Think about what will be useful to him in the long term. Does he need to modify his goals? Does he need to take smaller steps or does he need to dream bigger dreams?
2. Set long-term goals to keep your child progressing.
3. What does your child plan to do if her anxiety comes back?
4. What benchmarks can your child use to keep anxiety from taking over her life?
5. Have your child write a story, using the following outline, to celebrate her success in defeating the Dragon.

> My Story about How I Won Against the Dragon
>
>> Part 1: The characters
>>
>> Part 2: The situation
>>
>> Part 3: The problem
>>
>> Part 4: What I tried—what helped and what didn't help
>>
>> Part 5: What happened next

Part 6: What I learned

Part 7: What I plan to do if the Dragon comes back

Part 8: What I would like to tell another kid who has fears like mine

*Action Steps*

- Let the Dragon fade, but have a plan in case it returns.
- Remember the benefits of repeated praise. Give your child two compliments for every criticism.
- Help your child appreciate his own accomplishments in this major victory.

PART THREE

*Beyond Anxiety*

# CHAPTER 10

# Assessing Your Family's Role in Anxiety Disorders

Children who struggle with anxiety may feel isolated, thinking that no one understands what's happening to them. They have feelings other people don't have. They worry that other people, even their own parents, don't understand their anxious feelings. Although the Dragon speaks differently to each child, articulating that individual's worst fears, the Dragon's message is always the same: that the anxious child is alone with his suffering. The Dragon says that telling others will make the situation worse, because others will humiliate him. Yet those around the child who has an anxiety problem usually know that something is seriously wrong. The two most common signs that parents notice are a child's demands to do things in certain bizarre ways or the strangely quiet mood that overcomes him. Both a demanding, upset child and a quiet, withdrawn one will likely have a big impact on the family. It's useful to think of your family's role in coping with your child's anxiety problem, because the family team is the best defense against the Dragon. Families often change dramatically to enable an anxious child, in hopes of placating the Dragon. Yet families can channel these same feelings of wanting to help the child in a better direction, by putting the Dragon in its place.

I love to scare children by making them think that they can't tell their family members, who love them, how scared they really are. I say that adults don't understand how they feel and will make fun of them or punish them if they talk about what they experience.

We know a family with a two-year-old girl that took a trip to a city museum. While walking with her grandmother, the little girl suddenly noticed a sidewalk grate covering the underground drainage system. She could hear water dripping a long way down into the deep black hole. She looked up and was alarmed to see her mother was on the other side of the grate. She screamed and her mother ran to comfort her. Just as quickly, the girl's six-year-old brother playfully jumped on the grate to show her how strong it was. His excitement at this new city game, jumping on each grate as they walked down the street, made his little sister giggle. Without another hug from her mom, she picked up her brother's game and also began jumping on the grates. What could have been a moment of terror, resulting in a long-term traumatic memory, was suddenly transformed into a wonderful children's game.

Remember, there are valuable things to learn from fear. Fear itself, like the alarm of danger, is normal and healthy. Fear can keep a child safe—for example, by reminding him to wear a helmet every time he rides a bike. Tell your child that there are healthy, normal reasons to fear, and show him when you are afraid of real dangers, too.

Not every family or child will find a graceful way to avoid a moment of terror like this. In fact, many families won't even recognize clearly when such a moment occurs in their lives. Even more interesting, what would most families say about the six-year-old boy jumping on the grates? That he wasn't responding sensitively to his sister's terror, that he wasn't being careful himself, that the grates could be dangerous? This family had already spent many years battling the anxiety Dragon in multiple generations, so in one moment they had a flash of recognition that this was an opportunity to confront the Dragon, not to add unreasonable fears. The kids' mom reassured herself by saying that if the grates in the street were strong enough to hold her, they could surely hold a child jumping on them. The children's grandmother agreed. The family continued walking to the museum in good humor, rightly feeling that they had won an important victory. They had prevented a long-term problem and had some extra fun on their city adventure, as a result of the Dragon's unexpected appearance.

This family shows us a simple way to successfully handle an anxious moment. Though not nearly as complex and long-standing as many anxiety problems in this book, this example clearly shows the wonderful coping skills of a family that has worked as a team to handle anxiety. Start with thinking about the two-year-old first encountering what seems like a vast, deep, thoroughly scary hole in the sidewalk. It's important not to underestimate this little girl's fear—her terror was mixed with horror that such a thing could exist. While her mother empathized with the terror and rightly rushed to comfort her, her brother intuitively sensed that the best way to escape a moment of terror was to find humor in it. This isn't humor at the expense of the frightened person or humor that teases. Rather, it's fear that turns into fun, which is an important emotional catharsis in many successful books and movies. It's like

> Feared situations offer a choice: run, or learn how to cope and grow in the process of confronting them. Think of how many memorable situations in life require facing a fear and overcoming it. Unreasonable anxiety can be overwhelming, as well as inappropriate, but it also offers a great chance for growth for the anxious child and the whole family.

the ghost in the bedroom that, when the lights are turned on, is revealed to be a bathrobe over a chair, or the spooky noise that in reality is the neighbor's elderly dog trying to get in your back door.

One reason that families are able to use humor to overcome terror is that most families are founded on love and trust. This little girl loved and trusted her brother. She knew that he would show her the true situation, not the terror that she had imagined. Similarly, the mother and the grandmother trusted each other to decide that the children both were safe jumping on the grates. They also believed that no one had purposely caused the girl's fear. In a family that functions well, this moment-by-moment teamwork benefits everyone. It's possible to imagine many other outcomes if this family hadn't worked together constructively. The grandmother and the mother could have gotten angry with each other, or with the brother, for not being more sympathetic to the child's distress. Or the adults could have cautioned the son that unfamiliar city grates were dangerous, thus confirming the little girl's fears. One can also imagine the careful walk down the street they might have taken, with everyone avoiding grates for fear of further traumatizing the girl. That kind of avoidance, out of love and respect for the child's terribly distressing feelings, would almost inevitably have led her to be more deeply afraid of sidewalk grates than ever, and for good reason. The people she trusted most in her life had avoided something, so it must actually be dangerous. If the girl had been more frightened for her brother and worried that his life, too, might be in danger, the family would have had to move on to another coping strategy. The first approach doesn't always work, as it did in this happy example.

As you think about this story, imagine all of the members of your own family and the roles they play in enabling or trying to overcome your child's anxiety. Write each family member's name on an individual piece of paper, with a list below the name of the attitudes that person usually takes toward anxiety in his or her own life. Some people get angry, some sympathize, some look to others for help. The list of responses to anxiety is as varied as the families that struggle with this problem. Now, with all of your pieces of paper, try "walking" your family members down an unfamiliar city street like the one in the example. Who is scared of the grate? Who pulls the fearful person back from the grate? Who walks around the grates farther down the street? How do the other people in your family respond to this problem? In this example, it was a young child who was scared, but older children and adults can suddenly become scared of grates on a city sidewalk. What do you imagine would happen in your family?

If you were afraid of grates on a city sidewalk, what would you do? Having worked with thousands of anxious adults, we know the answer to that one: walk around the grates and tell no one you are afraid. Adults and older kids recognize that most of their anxious fears are unrealistic. They know that other people don't share these fears. Rather than confronting either their fears or the teasing of others, they keep their fears a secret and just avoid the problems in their lives every way they can. Most adults who fear driving on an interstate highway or flying, for example, don't want others to know this so they make thousands of apparently unrelated excuses for why they don't want to go someplace that requires them to travel on a big highway or in an airplane.

Researchers looking at the biological reason for anxiety in animals find that within a single species, individual animals (like dogs or cats) exhibit very different degrees of fear in the same situation. Although the fearless animals in a species may not live as long, they are often quicker to reproduce. In contrast, the more fearful animals in a species may live longer and therefore have a longer time over which to reproduce. Both anxiety and boldness are important qualities for survival of a species. (Dugatkin. *Cheating Monkeys and Citizen Bees: The Nature of Cooperation in Animals and Humans*, New York: Free Press, 1999)

Anger is a common reaction to anxiety. Sometimes the anxious child gets angry. Other times, the father does or, less frequently in our experience, the mother. Though it's normal and understandable to be frustrated by the limitations caused by a child's anxiety, remember that you can be angry at the anxiety problem and not at the anxious child. As one traditional father put it, "I would be angry if I thought my son was being disobedient to me, but I understand now that the OCD is talking at these times, so I find ways to handle the situation without anger instead of punishing him when he says 'no' to me." Just as we urge people to confront their unrealistic fears, so, too, we ask adults and kids to take responsibility for how they manage their anger. Anxiety problems can be lightning rods for anger. You may need to back away from the anxiety problem and address how anger is handled altogether in your family if you notice this problem reappearing. Consider getting help from a therapist or a clergy member if your family has trouble managing anger. It's a big problem for some people and thus for some families. It's best to handle anger problems straightforwardly by getting help. People need to realize that they can be angry without physically or emotionally hurting someone else.

Fear, of course, is not just about an unexpected grate in the sidewalk. Other fears are specific to certain children and families. A child with a chronic illness or whose parent is seriously ill may have realistic fears to face on a regular or irregular basis. Responding appropriately to these fear-generating situations can save someone's life, but they can also cause kids to feel constant anxiety—a heightened vigilance—that can make action in a scary situation more difficult.

When her two biological children and three adoptive children were old enough to recognize the numbers on the phone, a diabetic mother taught each child how to call 911 if she was unconscious. She knew that the smaller children might be home with her if she had a diabetic emergency and that they couldn't rely on the older children, who might be at school. Each child learned the correct steps to take and practiced carefully with the mother. Then they all showed each other that they knew how to do the right thing. The older kids applauded each child's passing the test, which proved that the child was a responsible member of the family and could help keep them all safe. This positive coping plan was needed one day when the mother was home with the youngest child, who had a profound learning disability. The mother passed out on the stairs. The child, despite being so terrified that she stuttered and couldn't say a full sentence to the 911 dispatcher, summoned help as she had learned to do. Though she was terribly frightened for her mother and scared at being left briefly with the neighbors when the ambulance took her mother to the hospital, the girl was confident in her role as the family hero. She knew how to do the right thing to save her mother's life. This child confronted her worst fear, and, as a result, her self-confidence grew.

Both of these examples show the importance of role-playing in confronting anxiety and in normalizing what is truly frightening. Role-playing means that adults think about what will likely be a hazard and how they want their children to cope with fearful situations. Every day parents act as an example of how to do things. The old adage "Do as I say, not as I do" is not helpful when coping with anxiety. Kids see what their parents are afraid of and how they handle their fears. Parents want to keep their kids safe but also want them to have the self-confidence to face a world with real risks. This self-confidence comes in part from knowing how to separate things that are truly dangerous from those that just appear to be dangerous. Parents can teach their children what to do in both situations. These lessons are important for parents to review as the world around them changes. Parents can also learn from their children what is truly frightening and what isn't. Notice that family learning goes two ways. Children can teach adults how to handle fears. Remember our story about the city sidewalk grate—it was the six-year-old who was the hero of that story.

*Action Steps*

- Model appropriate ways to handle new situations, with a mixture of caution and interest.
- Consider how anger is managed in your family. It's important for everyone to be able to get angry without hurting another person and without fear of being hurt.

# CHAPTER 11

# Anxiety, Terrorism, and Other Extraordinary Threats to Children

Parents often say that it's hard to raise children these days because life is so filled with dangers. The events of September 11, 2001, when terrorists took over four commercial airliners and turned them into suicide bombs, underscored this painful point. Terrorists showed no mercy to civilians, not even to children. The ongoing risks of new threats following the initial terrorist attacks in New York and Washington were even more disturbing because many parents worried that their families would be victimized by chemical, biological, or nuclear weapons of mass destruction. This is a classic "What if" fear. It's impossible to prevent anyone, including any particular child, from being victimized at any time. That is the formula for worry and anxiety. When doubt and uncertainty arise, fear can control an individual's feelings and behavior.

Who can forget the tragic events in Oklahoma City in 1995, when the destruction of the Alfred P. Murrah Federal Building by Timothy McVeigh killed more than one hundred federal workers, including every child in a busy day-care center on the building's ground floor? Children are not exempt from the dangers of modern life, much as we would like them to be. Children also face a multitude of more mundane risks, from gun violence to sexual abuse.

Violence at school has been a major fear of parents during the last few years.

> Talk with your child about risks—from automobile accidents and school violence to terrorism and bicycles. Talk about health risks, some of which can be controlled—like smoking cigarettes and using illegal drugs—while others are universal but generally uncontrollable, like asthma and leukemia. Help your child put these risks into perspective; help him see how he can reduce (but not eliminate) his risks. Let him know that you and other adults will be there to help him when he has problems.

Beyond these risks to children are the dangers of contracting serious illnesses, from genetic diseases like cystic fibrosis and diabetes, to fatal illnesses like cancer and heart disease. An even bigger threat is the risk of accidents, with automobile crashes leading the list. Children are definitely not safe in an absolute sense of the word. No amount of parental reassurance, however sincere, can ensure children's safety. The risks to children are serious, and no child is immune.

Not only are risks to children unevenly distributed in society, but fear is also unevenly distributed. With any particular risk—say, that of being on a flight hijacked by terrorists or the possibility of getting childhood leukemia—the fear engendered among the nation's children varies from crippling and constant to nonexistent. Equally uneven is the distribution of fear among American parents. Some parents are worried sick by risks their children face, while other parents don't give a thought to possible dangers that their children encounter every day.

So, there you have it. Dangers to children not only are real, but even the most conscientious parents cannot avoid them. Fear, like risk, is real for children. Surprisingly, the fears of both parents and children are not well connected to actual risks. Many children who are at high risk of encountering violence, accidents, or illness have little or no fear. At the same time, some children who, statistically, have a very low chance of harm coming to them nevertheless suffer from debilitating fears. When fear itself is a contagion in the community and the nation—as it was after the September 11 terrorist attacks—what can parents do, especially if their child has an anxiety problem? This question is even more complex when the parent also has an anxiety problem.

> Different children need different things from their parents. Naturally fearless children need their parents' help to learn to be more aware of risks. Naturally fearful children need their parents' help to put their risks into a more realistic perspective and not be imprisoned by their fears.

Let's begin by focusing on the risk part of the risk/fear/anxiety problem. We'll deal with the fear and the anxiety aspects after we understand risk. Until the last seventy years or so in the United States, the risk of death for a newborn child was about 20 percent before the age of five. This meant that in the nineteenth century and the early decades of the twentieth century, one-fifth of all American children were dead before their fifth birthdays. Today 99 percent of newborns reach the age of five in the United States. In the past, the death rate for children went down after the age of five but still remained high. Today, the chance of a child dying after the age of five is very small, on a statistical basis, but even today, the risk of children dying in childhood is not zero. Most children in the world—those who live in less-developed nations—have a very high risk of death, sometimes reaching 50 percent by the age of five. The risk of serious illnesses and handicaps for children has also fallen sharply in the United States and other economically developed nations during the last century. These dramatically falling childhood death rates happened for a reason. They are the result of improvements in health care, sanitation, and nutrition, as well as many other factors.

Remember, children have faced terrible risks for tens of thousands of years throughout human history. Parents and children have proven to be highly resilient, despite these terrible risks. If they hadn't been so resilient, our species wouldn't have survived, let alone thrived, as it clearly has.

When American parents lament the serious risks to children today, they seldom have this historical perspective. They aren't aware that their own children have a lower risk of death and serious illness than do children anywhere in the world, at any previous time. Even today, after the recent terrorist attacks, American children are among the safest and most secure of all the children in the world. In other words, although certain serious risks to children are relatively new in the developed world—such as automobile accidents—the overall serious health risks to children in the United States are at historically low levels.

> Your child needs to confront the sources of his anxieties gradually and repeatedly. You can help him do that and also help him feel good about this work.

In particular, the risks from terrorism are remarkably low for children (and for every other age group), not only in the United States but throughout the world. The 3,000 deaths resulting from the events of September 11 were devastating and unprecedented. Even when taking into account those terrible deaths, the risk of dying in the United States from terrorism remains small. It is striking that the deaths caused by the events of September 11 were without historical precedent. They compare with the more than 2,000 Americans killed in the December 7, 1941, attack on Pearl Harbor and the 3,700 Americans who died at the battle of Antietam during the American Civil War, the highest number of American casualties on any day of any war in the nation's history. The worst U.S. disasters before September 11, 2001, were the hurricane and the resulting flood in Galveston, Texas, in 1900; the 1906 earthquake and flood in San Francisco; and the fire in Chicago in 1876. None of those disasters produced more than 5,000 deaths.

Here's another perspective on the tragic death toll from September 11, 2001. On an average day about 8,000 Americans die. About 1,000 of them die as a result of smoking cigarettes and about 250 die, directly or indirectly, from drinking alcohol. This means that to reach the total of 3,000 Americans who died on September 11, 2001, as a result of terrorism, it takes three days of ordinary deaths from smoking and about two weeks of the deaths from alcohol consumption. Why do the deaths from terrorism so frighten us and why are other deaths—which occur day after day—so easily taken for granted?

> Use your support systems to help you deal with your fears, as well as those of your child. Teachers, pediatricians, family, friends, neighbors, therapists, and psychiatrists can all help.

Our nation is fortunate in its ability to provide health care and abundant resources for our children. Yet, paradoxically, over the last few decades we have become increasingly risk-averse, even as the actual risk to the health and safety of our children has fallen. To underscore this point, parents whose children are at relatively high risk often have a low degree of fear for their children, whereas parents whose children are at relatively low risk often feel high levels of fear.

In the United States we are bombarded by the media, which zero in on our fears like heat-seeking missiles tracking fighter jets. The ubiquitous media fan the flames of our fear. This doesn't happen because the various types of media are involved in a plot to distort or exaggerate our fears. The media put in front of us what we want to see, hear, and read. Our fear gets our attention, which in turn gets the attention of the media. We are part of a pernicious feedback loop, in which our fears encourage the media to focus on fear-generating material, and media attention to this fear-generating material further provokes our fears. The psychology of fear is well understood. What is familiar (like death from cigarette smoking) is not feared, despite its very real risk, yet an unfamiliar danger (like terrorist-spread anthrax or smallpox) is excessively feared.

> Children in America today are much safer than they were one hundred years ago. Yet children face risks we might not even consider: for example, choking while they eat or food poisoning. These risks are small but real. Instead of reacting emotionally to perceived risks, we should learn the facts about real risks so that our efforts can be directed toward actually keeping kids safe, instead of worrying over fairly small risks. (*Harvard Center for Risk Analysis*, vol. 8, no. 4 [April 2000])

Another important psychological factor in the generation of fear is the appearance of control. If we sense that we have control of a risk, we don't fear it. If we don't have personal control of a risk, we exaggerate that risk. This explains why so many people fear flying (an experience that is relatively unfamiliar to many people and a risk that they don't control) and feel so little fear driving an automobile (a familiar risk that most people think they do control). Yet these fears run counter to reality. Our risk is exceedingly low when flying and relatively high when driving. Typical parental fears for children are high when the child is flying and low when the parent is driving the child in a car. Thus, fear is not well correlated with actual risk for easily understood psychological reasons.

The media do not report cigarette-smoking deaths because we don't fear these. The media do not cover automobile fatalities because the risks from vehicular accidents are familiar. Terrorist threats are covered because we're unfamiliar with these and don't feel that we have control over risks that we face from terrorism.

Before we discuss fear and anxiety, let's review our findings about risk to children. It's important for parents to realize that their children are never safe in any absolute sense. Although risks to children in the United States are generally very low, there will always be some degree of risk. Parents need to talk honestly with their children about the risks they face and help them reduce their risks in prudent ways. For example, it's important for children to wear seatbelts when riding in automobiles and helmets when riding bikes or roller-blading on the street. Children shouldn't get into cars with strangers and should avoid using cigarettes, alcohol, and drugs. Beyond these basics of risk reduction, however, parents must help children accept the risks of everyday life in the United States. Parents should tell their children that they are safer than children have ever been before in history, and that if problems do develop, parents and many other caring people will help them. Everyone faces risks in life, both children and adults. That's how life is, how it always has been, and how it always will be. We must help our children understand their risks and how to reduce them, as well as how to cope with problems that develop.

Anthrax and smallpox—two unfamiliar, fatal diseases. You don't even know when you're exposed to them. They could hit anyone, anytime. No one knows for sure whether he is exposed or not. I can use those dangers to get parents and children into my prison—where they think they'll be safe from anthrax and smallpox.

Now let's discuss fear. Fear is good. It is healthy, helpful, and an appropriate reaction to real danger. What children need from adults, including parents, is help in identifying the dangers in their lives. Children need to know which things are sensible to fear and which are not. Parents can help with this categorizing, especially if they recognize that some children are naturally fearless while others are born fearful. The first group—the fearless kids—needs help in learning to fear what is truly dangerous. Fearful children need help in managing their fears when these fears are inappropriate.

Fearless kids need to remember to always wear seatbelts in cars and helmets while on their bikes. Fearful children must learn not to fear staying overnight at a friend's home or starting school in a new class with an unfamiliar teacher.

Beyond fears lie anxieties, persistent and repetitive patterns of fear that are inappropriate to the situations in which they occur. The anxiety is excessive in comparison to the actual risks faced by the child. Anxiety is a false alarm, a signal of danger when none exists. When dealing with terrorism and extraordinary threats, parents face the same problems that they do with more mundane fears. The best tactics to try will depend on what their particular children need. When managing fear and anxiety, one size does not fit all. Only customized solutions for one child at a time can succeed. Nevertheless, several important principles can provide guidance for parents and children. Children with anxiety problems often feel bad about their anxiety. They are aware that their peers, and often their siblings, don't have similar feelings. Parents need to help children understand the nature of their particular problem. They need to reassure the anxious child that his anxiety is a false alarm; the anxiety is distressing but not dangerous. Children need help in gradually and repeatedly confronting their fears. Anxious children need encouragement, support, respect, and love—especially when facing their fears.

Terrorism is my kind of problem. Everyone is scared and no one knows when and where the next disaster will occur. Even if months or years go by with no attacks, the fear seems reasonable. After all, no one knows the time or the place or even what the next crisis will be.

When parents have an anxiety problem, they usually know when their fears are excessive and when these are appropriate to the situations in which they occur. The easy way to tell the difference between reasonable fears and unreasonable anxieties is to see what normal people do in a similar situation. Anxious parents should then use that behavior as their own standard. For example, with fear of flying, parents with an anxiety problem need to "imperson-ate a normal person" while on a plane.

With terrorism and other unusual risks, sometimes an anxious parent doesn't know what's "normal" and what isn't. Fearful parents can sort that out by talking with people who are knowledgeable about the feared dangers. Here's an example of how this can work. A mother who was afraid of poison ivy had a son who, at the age of twelve, was unable to hike or camp with his friends because he feared getting poison ivy. Neither the mother nor the son had ever had poison ivy. Wherever they saw green things growing, they were certain that hidden in the foliage was the dreaded poison ivy. They both knew that other parents and other twelve-year-old kids didn't fear poison ivy the way they did. Their job together was to accept the risk of getting poison ivy. It is a real risk. They needed to accept that the boy could get poison ivy if he accompanied his friends into the woods. That risk could not be avoided. He truly might get poison ivy. But when the mother talked it over with her son's pediatrician, it was clear to both parent and child that the risk of getting poison ivy was manageable. Poison ivy is a treatable, nonfatal disease. For many years, this parent and this child had vastly exaggerated the risks of poison ivy. They were terrified of what is a minor and easily managed health problem. Their shared fear had crippled this boy for too long. It was important for them to confront their fears and work on exposing themselves to plants and to the chance of getting poison ivy. The mother needed to practice exposing herself as much as the son did. Doing the practice together helped them both.

> I work with human biology, not against it. I look for people with hair-trigger danger alarms built into their brains. All I have to do with these people is whisper in their ears, "Are you really sure there is no danger right now?" Their active imaginations do the rest for me.

That was an easy example because most people understand that the danger from poison ivy is relatively minor. Here's a harder one. A ten-year-old girl feared flying. She explained that the main thing she feared was the plane crashing. Her mother had not flown in a dozen years. She, too, had a fear of flying—or, more accurately, a fear of commercial airplanes crashing. It isn't too hard to convince a fearful mother and a fearful child that they could survive an attack of poison ivy. How could this family be convinced to overlook the relatively small risk of a plane crash? The child wasn't likely to survive a plane crash. Unlike poison ivy, a plane crash is often fatal. There was nothing they could do to mitigate the risk of the child's plane crashing. Wearing a seatbelt on an airplane is a good idea because it keeps you in your seat during air turbulence, but a seat belt is unlikely to make a plane crash survivable. The mother and her daughter reviewed the risks and learned that these were statistically low. But they said, quite correctly, "Our risks are not zero. No one knows which plane will crash and which one will arrive safely. Why risk a child's plane crashing if the child doesn't have to fly?" This logic kept the girl on the ground and out of airplanes. In a reversal of the advertising for the lottery ("You can't win if you don't play"), their logic went like this, "You can't crash if you don't fly!" What's wrong with seemingly sensible reasoning?

To answer this question, you have to think clearly about both the risks and the benefits of flying. The benefits were that the child could go places—like visit grandparents in a distant city—that, for practical purposes, were impossible without air travel. Beyond that benefit was the issue of how the child felt about herself and what her peers thought of her. When she didn't fly, she felt worse about herself. Her peers thought she was weak and strange. The risks of this girl's plane crashing truly were quite small, but they were not absolutely zero. In a bad year, up to 600 Americans die in commercial aircraft crashes. After 266 were killed in crashes on September 11, 2001, the number of people who died in aviation-related accidents during that year remained under 600 in the United States. In 2002 no one died in a plane crash in the United States. That risk is compared to the more than 3 million people who fly each day.

Those risks are so small, they make the odds of winning the lottery look good.

But what if parents and children fear a terrorist attack? What about the risks of bioterrorism? What about anthrax or smallpox or the agents from a rogue state exploding a nuclear device in an American city? Like the risks of flying, and unlike the risks of poison ivy, the consequences of a negative outcome in these circumstances are truly catastrophic. How likely are those catastrophic outcomes for any particular child? The answer is clear—they are very, very low. Lower even than the risks of airplane crashes. The risks to a child from terrorism are much smaller than the risk of having a fatal bicycle accident, for example. Automobiles are a much greater risk for children, both the risk of injury and that of death from their own family car.

But, you rightly ask, "Who is to say what the future holds?" No one can say that the future will not see tens of thousands or even hundreds of thousands of deaths from terrorism. This is a "What-if" nightmare. Just as no one can say that a particular child won't get leukemia or that a particular plane won't crash, no one can say that a particular child will not become a victim of terrorism.

To answer the question about what are reasonable risks for a child, whether from a bicycle or from anthrax, a caring parent not only needs to consider the likelihood of a catastrophic negative outcome but also needs to think about the costs of protective action. The cost of wearing a helmet when getting on a bike or wearing a seatbelt when riding in a car are so small as to be virtually negligible. The costs of not flying are not a matter of life and death, but they are substantial. By not flying, a child misses out on many valuable opportunities.

A woman in our practice reacted to the sixth case of anthrax in the United States by demanding of her husband that they take their three children out of school in Washington, D.C., and move to her family's home in the rural Midwest. The husband said, "No." He didn't think this was reasonable; the costs to the children would be too great. His wife, to put it bluntly, thought that he was putting their children's lives at risk.

This family's situation was made much worse because the parents were going through a painful divorce. Because of that stress, every decision they made turned into a major conflict. It's easy to see that the question of their children's safety wasn't a small problem. We suggested that this feuding couple focus on the best interests of the children, not on settling a score. We urged the parents to talk with their pediatrician about the children's best interests before making this life-changing decision. These children attended a prestigious private school. We suggested that the parents also talk with teachers and even the headmaster of the school, as well as with the parents of the children's best friends. After all, those parents faced the same problem, and many of them had the financial resources to move out of Washington if they decided this was the best course of action.

When all of the talking was done, the answer was clear, even to this anxious mother. Everyone was upset by the recent news about terrorism. Almost everyone in Washington worried that living in the nation's capital might add to the risks their children faced. These particular parents realized that their children were in a wonderful school and that although the risks of terrorism were not zero, they were reasonable to accept at this point. The parents also agreed that they might come to a different conclusion in the future, if the facts changed dramatically.

Bombs and hijacking are one kind of terrorism. Strange as it is to contemplate, those risks are relatively easy to deal with. They're like the risks of flying: either your plane crashes, or it doesn't. If you land, you know you're safe, although you have to deal with the next flight, and one safe arrival doesn't guarantee a similar outcome on the next flight. To some extent, the risks of bombs and hijacking are familiar, but terrorism engenders worse worries than hijacked jet planes. Anthrax, smallpox, and plagues are truly terrifying possibilities that can unnerve any parent or child. No one knows when or where the next terrorist attack will come. Unlike a crashing plane, with chemical, biological, and nuclear weapons, you can't be sure when your child is "hit" and when she is safe. When you see someone who looks suspicious, what should you do? What is "suspicious," anyway? Whatever is unfamiliar to us looks suspicious. We confront plenty of unfamiliar things every day. How many times do you see "white powder" in your life? How often do you get a letter from an unknown person or an unknown address? What about your child taking the subway, a train, or a trip to visit Capitol Hill or the White House, even when accompanied by a trusted adult? The "What if" dangers in these scenarios are limitless.

Our advice about these risks is clear and simple: accept that you and your child are vulnerable. Do whatever makes sense for you and your child. Turn to knowledgeable advisers when assessing risks and deciding how to protect your child. Your child's pediatrician and teachers can help. The police and other officials, including those at the Centers for Disease Control (CDC) and your local public health department, can also help. All of these people have expertise that you don't have. They are responsible for helping to protect you and your family from risks, including risks from terrorism. You can also benefit from talking with neighbors and the parents of your children's friends. You are not alone. Neither is your child. Take advantage of the support you have, and teach your child to recognize and use the help that is available.

When it comes to terrorism and other terrible (and unfamiliar) threats to your child, use the resources available to you to distinguish between risks that are reasonable to take and those that aren't. Playing in the woods (risking poison ivy) was a reasonable risk to take, considering the benefits for the boy we described. Riding a bike without a helmet is not a reasonable risk for a child to take. Flying on a commercial airplane is a reasonable risk. Teenage kids smoking cigarettes is not a reasonable risk. Living in Washington D.C., despite the continuing threats of terrorist attacks, is a reasonable risk, despite the possible unknown dangers.

If you recognize that your fears or your child's are beyond the limits of what is appropriate for a given situation, don't feel guilty and don't despair. Whether your child's anxiety problem is triggered by terrorism or by more ordinary things like the fear of having a panic attack or being exposed to "contamination," the techniques you both need to use are the same. The problem of anxiety does not exist outside the person. It is inside. Your child must overcome the real and certain danger of feeling discomfort, anxiety, and panic. The more your child can accept those bad feelings and act in a normal, ordinary way, the better off he is. The more he lets those bad feelings cripple him, the harder it becomes to reclaim his life.

*Action Steps*

- In your Journal, list your biggest fears for your child.
- Talk with friends, experts, and others about the risks faced by your child, as well as about your child's and your fears about these risks. Decide for yourself, but not by yourself, what's reasonable and what's not, regarding what you fear for your child.

CHAPTER 12

# Advice for Teachers, Coaches, Doctors, Therapists, School Nurses, and Others Who Work with Anxious Kids

Anxious children don't spend all of their time with their families. They also go to school, play on soccer teams, and participate in theater groups. Although this book was written primarily for parents of anxious children, we are frequently asked for advice by coaches and teachers who want to help excessively worried children. As a coach, a school nurse, or an involved adult volunteer, you often see anxious kids. You may not always know precisely what's going on with the child or even know that his problem is anxiety. Sometimes, you simply see the outward signs of distress, or else the kid doesn't show up for events that are considered fun, or at least manageable, by other kids.

We were in the process of writing this book when the events of September 11, 2001, overtook our country. Since then, there has been increased interest in how to help children and families cope with all types of fears. Fear affects everyone. One of the most difficult distinctions for a teacher or a volunteer scout leader to make is that between a reasonable and an unreasonable risk. Similarly, it can be tough to distinguish between a child with normal worries about real problems and a child who suffers from an anxiety problem. In earlier chapters of this book, you learned about the Dragon that scares kids by making them think that they have to do what the Dragon says, or else that mean Dragon will make bad things happen to children. The Dragon can produce strong, unpleasant physical sensations in the anxious child. You also learned about the Wizard, who teaches the child magic that can, in time, tame the Dragon. The scientist who wrote the Research Notes has also introduced himself and throughout the book has provided important scientific information about anxiety problems. You are in such an important position to help children that we want you to learn strategies to cope with anxiety problems as easily and as effectively as possible. The concept of the Wizard, the Dragon, and the Research Notes underlies all of our work. Therefore, we recommend that you go back and read Chapter 1 before proceeding. After you understand the Wizard, the Dragon, and the Research Notes, you can use this chapter on its own, without reading the rest of the book. Thank you for taking the time to learn more about helping anxious children.

Anxiety disorders are recognized as the most common mental health problem in the United States. Almost one in four people will have an anxiety disorder at some time in their lives. Combine this fact with the information that anxiety disorders start earlier in life than do other mental health problems, and you will realize that as an adult who works with young people, you are likely to meet kids who have anxiety problems. In each specific age group of children, it's amazing how many suffer from anxiety. An estimated 13 percent of children suffer from a diagnosable anxiety disorder. A far larger percentage of children occasionally suffer from anxiety problems like those described in this book. Working with a child who may have an anxiety problem is complicated for a teacher or coach. It's much easier if the parent tells you about it. Since there is still a stigma about mental health problems, it's understandable that some parents are not upfront with a coach or a volunteer church teacher about the diagnosis of a child's anxiety problem. We support the notion of privacy and of the parent and the child having the right to share only information that needs to be shared. It's important to respect this privacy. Nonetheless, however, you can still have a direct dialogue with the parent or the child about your group's specific expectations and goals. Then you, the parent, and the child can work together to achieve these goals. As a coach or a teacher, you are in a position to offer calm support and a safe environment for the child to learn to confront the anxiety Dragon.

It's important to make the distinction between normal anxiety, which is useful, and pathological anxiety, which is not. Everyone has normal anxiety from time to time. This consists of the heart beating fast and that "sweaty-hands feeling" we associate with taking a test or giving a talk to a group. This feeling focuses a child's attention as nothing else can. Anxiety helps children do their very best on the test or when giving a presentation. Pathological anxiety, in contrast to normal anxiety, is extreme and takes away from a child's concentration. Pathological anxiety interferes tremendously with daily life. It has a significant negative impact on one's daily functioning. These are not trivial or imperceptible problems. Anxiety disorders dominate the lives of most children who struggle with them.

Understanding that anxiety is not all or nothing is crucial to recovery. Try to think of anxiety as being on an ever-changing continuum; sometimes it's worse and sometimes it isn't so bad. Each anxiety episode may have different physical symptoms, and the symptoms may occur in different situations. Even so, it's crucial to understand that the overall intensity is actually quite variable, from minute to minute. We use a standard 0 to 10 scale to measure anxiety. Zero represents no anxiety; it is a calm, relaxed, productive state or a quiet resting state during sleep. Ten represents the worst panic a child ever had. This is usually the first panic attack, or one of the first, because the attacks are so new and the physical symptoms so worrisome that they tend to be the most extreme. Generally, anxiety after the first few attacks is always referenced back: "I'm afraid this will be as bad as that time at the play rehearsal." That time at play rehearsal was probably a Level 10.

Using a scale will help you have a meaningful dialogue with an anxious child without adding extra fear. You're not asking him to prove that he has a stomach ache or that his head hurts, but you're acknowledging his overall distress as it is measured on this 0 to 10 scale. A Level 7 of anxiety sounds more like a science experiment. Most kids do well pretending to be a scientist of their anxiety. Anxiety levels change quickly. Often, just stopping and waiting when anxiety is very high is an effective technique. A child may want to know that she can leave a situation if she needs to, but she will likely find the courage to stay if she knows that possibility is available. Anxiety generally goes down just from waiting a few minutes. That realization is reassuring to an anxious child. She needs to learn that she doesn't have to do anything to get the anxiety level to go down, except wait and let it fall on its own. Usually, talking with someone also brings her anxiety level down, especially if the other person knows about her anxiety problem.

One question that many teachers and coaches ask is how to distinguish between children who are trying to get attention or are in need of discipline and a child with an anxiety problem. This distinction can be tricky. Most people who teach children have at times thought that an anxious child was just misbehaving or being manipulative. The distinction is easier to make if you think through what the child is getting from the abnormal behavior. Most kids with anxiety disorders are clearly in acute distress when they have to confront something they are afraid of. They may be forced to do it anyway, but they are obviously struggling with overwhelmingly painful emotions. In contrast, kids who are motivated by getting attention or being able to spend a day home from school playing computer games will gain something obvious from their abnormal behavior. This may at times seem confusing, but if you think about our recommendations for recovery, you'll see that regardless of the reason for their reluctance, we ask kids to slowly and consistently face their fears. This generally separates kids who are motivated to get well from those who are not.

Feelings of anxiety are so overwhelming that most anxious kids are relieved and grateful to discover a way to get better. Although they might not like every step on the path, from the moment they understand that this method will help, their hope helps them take their first difficult steps. Perhaps you have an ongoing concern that a child is manipulating you or faking distress in order to get what he wants. We suggest that you try our approach, anyway. If it doesn't work, you'll have a record of what happened to use when you talk to the child's parent, the school psychologist, or your supervisor.

> I call anxiety a "disease of quality people." Children who worry tend to be conscientious and follow rules. They generally respect adults and work hard to meet their responsibilities, such as doing their homework. Anxious children may "misbehave" if the Dragon makes them feel bad, but they don't misbehave in order to get something special or to avoid doing chores. They might refuse to go to school to avoid panic but not to avoid being tested on their homework.

Helping children overcome serious and potentially disabling anxiety problems has rewards for you, as a coach or a group leader, that you might not see immediately. You have the opportunity to watch anxious children who were once controlled by anxiety suddenly blossom—free to be themselves, without limitations. This is a tremendous experience. It shows you, as nothing else can, that the children weren't just pretending to be distressed to get attention, but that they suffered from a real problem.

Anxiety represents a false alarm of danger. It is how a particular child's brain functions. These are normal feelings, but the Dragon makes the child feel them in inappropriate situations. The Dragon makes an anxious child fear things that don't frighten other children. The good news is that as a child learns to face the Dragon, with the help of the Wizard's magic, he will actually change his brain chemistry, so that after he is well, his brain will signal danger normally. His brain is no longer trapped by pathological anxiety in cycles of worried thought. Recovering from an anxiety problem is a tremendously powerful experience of positive change for a child.

As an adult who works with children, you can give a child no bigger gift than a new way of thinking or acting that will help him throughout his life. Be sure to appreciate the growth and the effort that this child has put into meeting his goals.

Respect the Dragon and the powerful feelings it generates in the anxious child. Yet respecting the Dragon doesn't mean giving in to the Dragon's demands. You should understand that battling the Dragon is painfully hard for an anxious child. Be sure to praise the child for his efforts, however small. This reinforcement will build self-confidence and encourage further efforts.

This experience of confronting inappropriate but terribly painful anxiety gives you an opportunity to rethink your own behavior and thoughts, too. Not only kids can set goals and change! By taking time to read this book, you have set a goal of learning more about anxiety and you have met that goal. Now you face the next goal—trying new techniques with the anxious child in your group. To begin this work, set up a folder with a page that lists what you have noticed to be this child's problems. Be as specific, yet as brief, as you can. List dates and situations. Describe what happened next. A chart format works well for this kind of record. Set up four columns as shown on page 197.

Do you notice any patterns to these problems? Do they always occur at the beginning of your meeting or at a stressful moment? Keep this chart going, as you change how you relate to this anxious child, to learn which techniques help.

Start a new page with your definition of the problem. Keep in mind that you are responding to the problem only as you see it, which may be quite different from how the child sees it. For example, it's a problem for you and the group if a child is so shy, she won't ever speak up in a church school class. It's also a problem if a child cries when his mother drops him off at soccer practice, or

| Date | Situation | What Happened | What Helped |
|------|-----------|---------------|-------------|
|      |           |               |             |
|      |           |               |             |
|      |           |               |             |
|      |           |               |             |
|      |           |               |             |
|      |           |               |             |

if a child won't do a Scouting project because he thinks that touching glue might hurt him. These are not rewarding moments for teachers or volunteer leaders. On the other hand, they are clearly unpleasant for the child as well. Reacting to your feeling of frustration, which may easily turn to anger, is likely to upset the child even further and lower his already shaky self-esteem. So, what can you do?

I overwhelm many anxious children with horrible physical feelings like stomach aches, sweating, and trembling. I'm an expert at making a worried child have these scary physical feelings. The bad feelings are not imaginary or made-up. I'm tricking the child by making these feelings happen at an inappropriate time and setting and by implying that these feelings will get worse and worse, leading to serious physical illness, passing out, or even death. Who can say that the bad feelings are "only anxiety"? Maybe this time they indicate a brain tumor or the first signs of leukemia.

Now that you have identified the problem behavior clearly, list your goals for this child. For example, with a shy child, you probably wouldn't start with a goal of her being the group leader. But you could talk to her about a goal of volunteering one brief comment in a class. For a child who cries when his mother leaves, you could set a goal of his not crying in front of his teammates unless he is injured. For the child who won't touch glue, you could set a goal that the child participate in all activities and projects so that he can collect badges along with his pack.

Wishes may come true on their own, but not for an anxious child. For that child, it takes work to feel well. The next step in making these goals a reality is to share them with the anxious child. You're offering the child an opportunity to learn to do something better than he has before. You're also asking him to make an important change in his behavior and his thinking. This will likely be a private conversation you have with the child. You may want his parents to participate as well. Whether you talk to the parents about your expectations, prior to talking to the child, depends on the specific situation and on how motivated the child is to participate. You don't want your goals and expectations to be a barrier to the child's participation. Rather, you will want to use the motivation the child has to be with the group as a source of strength for him as he confronts the Dragon. The fact that he is struggling with anxiety enough for you to notice his behavior problems means that he will likely be relieved that you have new ideas he can try to get well. Be calm, practical, and supportive. Remember that the Dragon speaks with menace and control, while the Wizard offers sympathetic rational choices. Whenever you can, speak in the Wizard's voice.

Your next page in the file about this child will be a list of options for you both to try, as you work together toward your shared goal. These choices may be either simple or complex. They could involve other kids in the group (without the kids knowing that they are helpers!) or they could involve you or the child's parent. The options will all involve the anxious child, however, so be sure to include him as you brainstorm new ways to handle this problem.

In the past, researchers didn't think that children younger than school-aged could benefit from cognitive restructuring. Recent research, however, shows that even very young children can have anxiety problems and can benefit from help in coping with them. This work with a young child will likely involve play or modeling new behaviors. An anxious two-year-old can benefit from hearing stories about kids who cope well with situations or from using puppets to put on a play about a frightening situation that has a happy ending. ("Effective CBT Targets Toddler's Cognitive Level," *Clinical Psychiatry News* [January 2002]: 36)

For example, the child who cries when his mother drops him off at soccer may dream of being a goalie. Why not create a reward system with him? Tell him that if he can walk to the field without crying, you will immediately set up a drill in which he is the goalie and the rest of the team lines up to practice, dribbling and passing the ball to shoot against him. This will probably be enough incentive, and sufficiently distracting, that he will be able to let his mother go with less outward distress. You may wonder if this will spoil the child. Keep in mind, this is a child who is clearly suffering, who wants to be on the team, and who needs extra help in doing so. Just as you would set up an extra drill to help a child with left-footed passing and then have all the kids on the team practice so that you didn't single that kid out, the same is true for this goalie exercise. If other kids protest that they want to be the goalie, too, then sometime during practice, you can spontaneously assign another kid to be goalie and have all the kids dribble and shoot against him.

This example illustrates how your flexibility can work well in confronting anxiety. Another way to think about the child's recovery process is that you have to be able to use what you have from the kids at any given time to teach them effectively. If a child wants to stay on the team, you don't want anxiety to prevent him from doing so. Although this method of dealing directly with a child's anxiety is more work than if you ignored the problem, it is also less distressing for you. It is definitely less distressing for the anxious child to begin working on his painful, disabling problem.

> Show consideration for a parent and a child who don't share information with you, if you think they have an anxiety problem. You can do a lot to help them even without this information, if you focus on your goals for this child. If they do share sensitive information with you, please respect their privacy unless they say that this information is public knowledge.

What about a situation where an anxious child or his parent asks you to make a special exception for him because the expectations you have for the other kids are too hard for him? You clearly don't want to give in to requests like this, which seem to allow the child to avoid the Dragon. On the other hand, making temporary adjustments can be fine. This shows the parents and the child that the Dragon can be confronted slowly and deliberately, with help from other people. Think about this in the context of the boy who wouldn't complete a Scouting project because he was afraid the glue would make him sick. Your goal is for him to do all of the projects and activities so that he can collect badges along with his pack. However, he may need to know ahead of time which projects will be done and have a parent volunteer to come along, while also bringing medication in case the activity is too anxiety-provoking. Or perhaps the group project of cleaning trash from a local park is overwhelming, despite his wearing gloves like the other kids. He could instead be the person who records on a clipboard how much trash is gathered, or the one who passes out clean trash bags. Eventually, it's important for him to participate fully in the activity. If, however, you make allowances for him to have an "out," a way to be part of the group without having to confront the Dragon at too high an anxiety level in front of his friends, this may be a way for him to eventually reach the goal of full participation. An "out" is a break from the Dragon. It is a Wizard trick that allows someone to keep working on a situation while taking a break from the intensity of the anxiety. An "out" is always better than running away from the Dragon, because running away makes the Dragon so much stronger the next time the child confronts the anxiety-provoking situation.

> I'm always looking for an opportunity to scare an anxious child by telling him he is trapped and alone. How can he be alone on a team or in a class, you ask? Just look at the anxious kid—he believes that no one understands him and no one will help him with this problem. And I just tell him that he's right. If you speak like the Wizard and help him calm down, it will wreck all my plans to have power over him!

Remember, the fundamental place to confront anxiety is in the child's mind. The anxious child has to do that work. You can and should encourage him and offer advice. Be his biggest cheerleader. Yet you can't solve his anxiety problem. You can do a lot, but the solution, like the problem, lies inside his mind. At first, that may seem unfair. Once you both accept that fact and the child starts to solve the problem, it will become obvious that the anxiety Dragon has given you both a gift. By confronting so formidable a problem, the child sets a positive model for his entire life. He acknowledges the problem, gets help to understand it, and then works hard to overcome it. This is a great gift indeed, and you can participate in the process.

### Action Steps

- Set up a chart to record anxiety problems as they occur with a particular child.
- Establish practical, achievable goals for the anxious child.
- Enlist the child's help in finding strategies that she can use to achieve these goals.

APPENDIX

# Diagnostic Criteria for Anxiety Disorders
## (from the *DSM-IV*)

I.  Criteria for Panic Attack

A discrete period of intense fear or discomfort, in which four (or more) of the following symptoms developed abruptly and reached a peak within 10 minutes:

    (1) palpitations, pounding heart, or accelerated heart rate

    (2) sweating

    (3) trembling or shaking

    (4) sensations of shortness of breath or smothering

    (5) feeling of choking

    (6) chest pain or discomfort

    (7) nausea or abdominal distress

    (8) feeling dizzy, unsteady, lightheaded, or faint

    (9) derealization (feelings of unreality) or depersonalization (being detached from oneself)

    (10) fear of losing control or going crazy

    (11) fear of dying

    (12) paresthesias (numbness or tingling sensations)

    (13) chills or hot flashes

II.  Diagnostic Criteria for 300.02 Generalized Anxiety Disorder

    A.  Excessive anxiety and worry (apprehensive expectation), occurring more days than not for at least 6 months, about a number of events or activities (such as work or school performance).

B. The person finds it difficult to control the worry.

C. The anxiety and worry are associated with three (or more) of the following six symptoms (with at least some symptoms present for more days than not for the past 6 months). **Note:** Only one item is required in children.

   (1) restlessness or feeling keyed up or on edge

   (2) being easily fatigued

   (3) difficulty concentrating or mind going blank

   (4) irritability

   (5) muscle tension

   (6) sleep disturbance (difficulty falling or staying asleep, or restless unsatisfying sleep)

D. The focus of the anxiety and worry is not confined to features of an Axis I disorder, e.g., the anxiety or worry is not about having a panic attack (as in panic disorder), being embarrassed in public (as in social phobia), being contaminated (as in obsessive-compulsive disorder), being away from home or close relatives (as in separation anxiety disorder), gaining weight (as in anorexia nervosa), having multiple physical complaints (as in somatization disorder), or having a serious illness (as in hypochondriasis), and the anxiety and worry do not occur exclusively during posttraumatic stress disorder.

E. The anxiety, worry, or physical symptoms cause clinically significant distress or impairment in social, occupational, or other important areas of functioning.

F. The disturbance is not due to the direct physiological effects of a substance (e.g., a drug of abuse, a medication) or a general medical condition (e.g., hyperthyroidism) and does not occur exclusively during a mood disorder, a psychotic disorder, or a pervasive developmental disorder.

III. Diagnostic Criteria for 309.81 Posttraumatic Stress Disorder

A. The person has been exposed to a traumatic event in which both of the following were present:

   (1) the person experienced, witnessed, or was confronted with an event or events that involved actual or threatened death or

serious injury, or a threat to the physical integrity of self or others

(2) the person's response involved intense fear, helplessness, or horror. **Note:** In children, this may be expressed instead by disorganized or agitated behavior

B. The traumatic event is persistently reexperienced in one (or more) of the following ways:

(1) recurrent and intrusive distressing recollections of the event, including images, thoughts, or perceptions. **Note:** In young children, repetitive play may occur in which themes or aspects of the trauma are expressed

(2) recurrent distressing dreams of the event. **Note:** In children, there may be frightening dreams without recognizable content

(3) acting or feeling as if the traumatic event were recurring (includes a sense of reliving the experience, illusions, hallucinations, and dissociative flashback episodes, including those that occur on awakening or when intoxicated). **Note:** In young children, trauma-specific reenactment may occur

(4) intense psychological distress at exposure to internal or external cues that symbolize or resemble an aspect of the traumatic event

(5) physiological reactivity on exposure to internal or external cures that symbolize or resemble an aspect of the traumatic event

C. Persistent avoidance of stimuli associated with the trauma and numbing of general responsiveness (not present before the trauma), as indicated by three (or more) of the following:

(1) efforts to avoid thoughts, feelings, or conversations associated with the trauma

(2) efforts to avoid activities, places, or people that arouse recollections of the trauma

(3) inability to recall an important aspect of the trauma

(4) markedly diminished interest or participation in significant activities

(5) feeling of detachment or estrangement from others

(6) restricted range of affect (e.g., unable to have loving feelings)

(7) sense of a foreshortened future (e.g., does not expect to have a career, marriage, children, or a normal life span)

D. Persistent symptoms of increased arousal (not present before the trauma), as indicated by two (or more) of the following:

(1) difficulty falling or staying asleep

(2) irritability or outbursts of anger

(3) difficulty concentrating

(4) hypervigilance

(5) exaggerated startle response

E. Duration of the disturbance (symptoms in Criteria B, C, and D) is more than 1 month.

F. The disturbance causes clinically significant distress or impairment in social, occupational, or other important areas of functioning.

*Specify* if:

**Acute:** if duration of symptoms is less than 3 months

**Chronic:** if duration of symptoms is 3 months or more

*Specify* if:

**with delayed onset:** if onset of symptoms is at least 6 months after the stressor

IV. Diagnostic Criteria for 300.3 Obsessive-Compulsive Disorder

A. Either obsessions or compulsions:

*Obsessions as defined by (1), (2), (3), and (4):*

(1) recurrent and persistent thoughts, impulses, or images that are experienced, at some time during the disturbance, as intrusive and inappropriate and that cause marked anxiety or distress

(2) the thoughts, impulses, or images are not simply excessive worries about real-life problems

(3) the person attempts to ignore or suppress such thoughts, impulses, or images, or to neutralize them with some other thought or action

(4) the person recognizes that the obsessional thoughts, impulses, or images are a product of his or her own mind (not imposed from without as in thought insertion)

*Compulsions as defined by (1) and (2):*

(1) repetitive behaviors (e.g., hand washing, ordering, checking) or mental acts (e.g., praying, counting, repeating words silently) that the person feels driven to perform in response to an obsession, or according to rules that must be applied rigidly

(2) the behaviors or mental acts are aimed at preventing or reducing distress or preventing some dreaded event or situation; however, these behaviors or mental acts either are not connected in a realistic way with what they are designed to neutralize or prevent or are clearly excessive

B. At some point during the course of the disorder, the person has recognized that the obsessions or compulsions are excessive or unreasonable. **Note:** This does not apply to children.

C. The obsessions or compulsions cause marked distress, are time consuming (take more than 1 hour a day), or significantly interfere with the person's normal routine, occupational (or academic) functioning, or usual social activities or relationships.

D. If another Axis I disorder is present, the content of the obsessions or compulsions is not restricted to it (e.g., preoccupation with food in the presence of an eating disorder; hair pulling in the presence of trichotillomania; concern with appearance in the presence of body dysmorphic disorder; preoccupation with drugs in the presence of a substance use disorder; preoccupation with having a serious illness in the presence of hypochondriasis; preoccupation with sexual urges or fantasies in the presence of a paraphilia; or guilty ruminations in the presence of major depressive disorder).

E. The disturbance is not due to the direct physiological effects of a substance (e.g., a drug of abuse, a medication) or a general medical condition.

*Specify* if:

**with poor insight:** if, for most of the time during the current episode, the person does not recognize that the obsessions and compulsions are excessive or unreasonable

V. Diagnostic Criteria for 300.23 Social Phobia

A. A marked and persistent fear of one or more social or performance situations in which the person is exposed to unfamiliar people or to possible scrutiny by others. The individual fears that he or she will act in a way (or show anxiety symptoms) that will be humiliating or embarrassing. **Note:** In children, there must be evidence of the capacity for age-appropriate social relationships with familiar people and the anxiety must occur in peer settings, not just in interactions with adults.

B.  Exposure to the feared social situation almost invariably provokes anxiety, which may take the form of a situationally bound or situationally predisposed panic attack. **Note:** In children, the anxiety may be expressed by crying, tantrums, freezing, or shrinking from social situations with unfamiliar people.

C.  The person recognizes that the fear is excessive or unreasonable. **Note:** In children, this feature may be absent.

D.  The feared social or performance situations are avoided or else are endured with intense anxiety or distress.

E.  The avoidance, anxious anticipation, or distress in the feared social or performance situation(s) interferes significantly with the person's normal routine, occupational (academic) functioning, or social activities or relationships, or there is marked distressed about having the phobia.

F.  In individuals under age 18 years, the duration is at least 6 months.

G.  The fear or avoidance is not due to the direct physiological effects of a substance (e.g., a drug of abuse, a medication) or a general medical condition and is not better accounted for by another mental disorder (e.g., panic disorder with or without agoraphobia, separation anxiety disorder, body dysmorphic disorder, pervasive developmental disorder, or schizoid personality disorder).

H.  If a general medical condition or another mental disorder is present, the fear in criterion A is unrelated to it, e.g., the fear is not of stuttering, trembling in Parkinson's disease, or exhibiting abnormal eating behavior in anorexia nervosa or bulimia nervosa.

*Specify* if:

**Generalized:** if the fears include most social situations (also consider the additional diagnosis of avoidant personality disorder)

VI. Diagnostic Criteria for 300.29 Specific Phobia

A.  Marked and persistent fear that is excessive or unreasonable, cued by the presence or anticipation of a specific object or situation (e.g., flying, heights, animals, receiving an injection, seeing blood).

B. Exposure to the phobic stimulus almost invariably provokes an immediate anxiety response, which may take the form of a situationally bound or situationally predisposed panic attack. **Note:** In children, the anxiety may be expressed by crying, tantrums, freezing, or clinging.

C. The person recognizes that the fear is excessive or unreasonable. **Note:** In children, this feature may be absent.

D. The phobic situation(s) is avoided or else is endured with intense anxiety or distress.

E. The avoidance, anxious anticipation, or distress in the feared situation(s) interferes significantly with the person's normal routine, occupational (or academic) functioning, or social activities or relationships, or there is marked distress about having the phobia.

F. In individuals under age 18 years, the duration is at least 6 months.

G. The anxiety, panic attacks, or phobic avoidance associated with the specific object or situation are not better accounted for by another mental disorder, such as obsessive-compulsive disorder (e.g., fear of dirt in someone with an obsession about contamination), posttraumatic stress disorder (e.g., avoidance of stimuli associated with a severe stressor), separation anxiety disorder (e.g., avoidance of school), social phobia (e.g., avoidance of social situations because of fear of embarrassment), panic disorder with agoraphobia without history of panic disorder.

*Specify* type:

**animal type**

**natural environment type** (e.g., heights, storms, water)

**blood, injection, injury type**

**situational type** (e.g., airplanes, elevators, enclosed places)

**other type** (e.g., phobic avoidance of situation that may lead to choking, vomiting or contracting an illness; in children, avoidance of loud sounds or costumed characters)

VII. Criteria for Agoraphobia

A. Anxiety about being in places or situations from which escape might be difficult (or embarrassing) or in which help may not be available in the event of having an unexpected or situationally predisposed panic attack or panic-like symptoms. Agoraphobic fears typically involve characteristic clusters of situations that include being outside the home alone; being in a crowd or standing in a line; being on a bridge; and traveling in a bus, train, or automobile.

**Note:** Consider the diagnosis of specific phobia if the avoidance is limited to one or only a few specific situations, or social phobia if the avoidance is limited to social situations.

B.  The situations are avoided (e.g., travel is restricted) or else are endured with marked distress or with anxiety about having a panic attack or panic-like symptoms, or require the presence of a companion.

C.  The anxiety or phobic avoidance is not better accounted for by another mental disorder, such as social phobia (e.g., avoidance limited to social situations because of fear of embarrassment), specific phobia (e.g., avoidance limited to a single situation like elevators), obsessive-compulsive disorder (e.g., avoidance of dirt in someone with an obsession about contamination), posttraumatic stress disorder (e.g., avoidance of stimuli associated with a severe stressor), or separation anxiety disorder (e.g., avoidance of leaving home or relatives).

VIII.   Diagnostic Criteria for 300.21 Panic Disorder with Agoraphobia

A.  Both (1) and (2):

(1)  recurrent unexpected panic attacks

(2)  at least one of the attacks has been followed by 1 month (or more) of one (or more) of the following:

(a)  persistent concern about having additional attacks

(b)  worry about the implications of the attack or its consequences (e.g., losing control, having a heart attack, "going crazy")

(c)  a significant change in behavior related to the attacks

B.  The presence of agoraphobia.

C.  The panic attacks are not due to the direct physiological effects of a substance (e.g., a drug of abuse, a medication) or a general medical condition (e.g., hyperthyroidism).

D.  The panic attacks are not better accounted for by another mental disorder, such as social phobia (e.g., occurring on exposure to feared social situations), specific phobia (e.g., on exposure to a specific phobic situation), obsessive-compulsive disorder (e.g., on exposure to dirt in someone with an obsession about contamination), posttraumatic stress disorder (e.g., in response to stimuli associated with a severe stressor), or separation anxiety disorder (e.g., in response to being away from home or close relatives).

# GLOSSARY

**Anticipatory anxiety**  Anticipatory anxiety is the anxiety experienced in anticipation of dreaded situations or experiences.

**Anxiety**  The threatening feeling of internal anxiety is one of the truly painful feelings that anxiety produces. Worry, tension, and irritability are usually part of the picture of anxiety.

**Agoraphobia**  Agoraphobia is the fear of being away from a safe person or a safe place.

**Cognitive-behavioral therapy (CBT)**  A new form of psychological treatment involving changing thoughts and behaviors with a lot of practice.

**The Dragon**  The Dragon is an imaginary creature that lives in an anxious child's mind and uses fear and unpleasant physical feelings of panic to control the child.

**Fear**  Fears are appropriate concerns about a danger considered to be a threat by most people. The fear reaction is helpful because it keeps the child safe.

**Generalized anxiety disorder (GAD)**  In generalized anxiety disorder, the worry is about multiple experiences and threats and is not focused on any one object or situation or associated with a specific behavior such as avoidance or a compulsion.

**Nervous**  This is a common term for anxious or worried.

**Obsessive-compulsive disorder (OCD)**  Obsessions are unwanted, unpleasant thoughts that get stuck in the anxious person's mind unless he

213

performs compulsions—ritualized, mindless activities. Often, OCD focuses on a fear of harming someone without wanting to.

**Panic attack**   A panic attack is a severe activation of a normal biological process that alerts your body to the presence of danger. Panic attacks occur when this activation is unrelated to real, immediate danger and instead happens either in specific situations, often leading to phobias, or out of the blue, in spontaneous panic attacks.

**Panic disorder**   Panic disorder is diagnosed when a person has repeated severe panic attacks that are painful and crippling. Panic disorder often leads to agoraphobia.

**Phobia**   A phobia is an inappropriate fear of a particular object or experience that leads to anxiety and avoidance of that object or situation.

**Psychiatrist**   A medical doctor specializing in the treatment of mental disorders.

**Practice**   To repeatedly and voluntarily put oneself in anxiety-provoking situations so the anxiety reaction diminishes.

**Situational panic attacks**   Situational panic attacks occur in generally predictable places or experiences, often worst in the absence of a safe person.

**Social anxiety disorder (SAD)**   Formally, social phobia. People with SAD fear embarrassment. This can lead to avoidance of social encounters, failure to make friends, and restriction of social activities, ranging from giving a speech to speaking up in class or even meeting or talking with strangers or people in authority.

**Specific phobic disorder**   Specific phobic disorder is the classic one-cause phobia, such as a fear of dogs or spiders, claustrophobia, or a fear of flying, without the features of agoraphobia or panic disorder.

**Spontaneous panic attacks**   Panic attacks that occur unpredictably, out of the blue, are spontaneous panic attacks.

**Therapist**   A psychologist, social worker, or other counselor who treats mental disorders.

**The Wizard**   The Wizard is an imaginary person who exists in an anxious child's mind. The Wizard offers children and their parents practical magic to tame the Dragon.

**Worry machine**   An imaginary machine in the anxious child's mind that churns out one worry after another.

# SUGGESTED ADDITIONAL READING

**Books for Kids**

Crary, E. *I'm Scared*. Seattle, Wash.: Parenting Press, Inc., 1996.

Crary, E. *Mommy, Don't Go*. Washington: Parenting Press, Inc., 1996.

Foster, C. *Kids Like Me: Children's Stories about Obsessive Compulsive Disorder*. Ellsworth, Maine: Solvay Pharmaceuticals, Inc., 1997.

Henkes, K. *Wemberly Worried*. Hong Kong: Greenwillow Books, 2000.

Porter, D. J., and C. Nathan. *Taming Monster Moments*. Mahwah, N.J.: Paulist Press, 1999.

**Books for Parents**

Chanskey, T. *Freeing Your Child from Obsessive-Compulsive Disorder*. New York: Times Books, 2000.

Dacey, J., and L. Fiore. *Your Anxious Child*. New York: John Wiley & Sons, 2000.

*Diagnostic and Statistical Manual of Mental Disorders, Fourth Edition, Text Revision*. Washington, D.C.: American Psychiatric Association, 2000.

Manassis, K. *Keys to Parenting Your Anxious Child*. Hauppauge, N.Y.: Barron's Educational Series, Inc., 1996.

Schneier, F., and Welkowitz, L. *The Hidden Face of Shyness*. New York: Avon Books, 1996.

*Special Focus on Anxiety Disorders in Children, Adolescents and Young Adults*. Rockville, Md.: Anxiety Disorders Association of America, 1998.

Stein, D. J., and E. Hollander, Eds. *Textbook of Anxiety Disorders*. Washington, D.C.: American Psychiatric Publishing, Inc., 2002.

# ANXIETY DISORDERS RESOURCES FOR PARENTS AND CHILDREN

## ADD Resources

Attention Deficit Disorder Association
P.O. Box 972
Mentor, OH 44061
(800) 487-2282
http://www.add.org

Children and Adults with Attention Deficit Disorders (CHADD)
499 Northwest Seventieth Avenue, Suite 308
Plantation, FL 33317
(305) 587-3700
http://www.chadd.org

## Anxiety Resource

Anxiety Disorders Association of America (ADAA)
11900 Park Lawn Drive, Suite 100
Rockville, MD 20852
(301) 231-9350
www.adaa.org

## Behavioral Problem Resource

Toughlove International
P.O. Box 1069
Doylestown, PA 18901
(215) 348-7090
www.toughlove.org

# Mental Health Resources

National Alliance for the Mentally Ill—Children
  and Adolescents Network (NAMICAN)
200 North Glebe Road, Suite 1015
Arlington, VA 22203
(800) 950-6264
www.nami.org

National Institute of Mental Health
NIMH Public Inquiries
6001 Executive Blvd., Rm. 8184 MSC 9663
Bethesda, MD 20892
(301) 443-4513
www.nimh.gov/home.cfm

# Obsessive Compulsive Resource

Obsessive-Compulsive Foundation
337 Notch Hill Rd.
North Branford, CT 06471
(203) 315-2190
www.ocfoundation.org

# Tourette's Syndrome Resource

Tourette Syndrome Association, Inc.
42-40 Bell Boulevard
Bayside, NY 11361
(718) 224-2999
www.tsa-usa.org

# INDEX

escitalopram (Lexapro), 72
exercise, 123–126, 144
exposure and response prevention,
    150–151
extended release alprazolam (Xanax
    XR), 71
extracurricular activities, 125–126,
    162

family team strategy, 53–54, 56,
    169–175. *See also* parents
fear, 2–3, 10, 24, 171, 213. *See also*
    phobias; risk; specific phobia
  age-appropriate, 24
  appropriate response to, 173–174
  of attention, 143–146
  of closed doors, 146–148
  of contamination, 115–117,
      148–151
  of dental work, 147
  of flying, 182, 186–187
  of harming self/others, 40
  level of, 88
  media and, 181–182
  of needles, 103–105
  patterns of, 184
  of poison ivy, 185
  reasonable, 184–185, 187, 189, 191
  of separation, 97
fearless children, 183–184
fight-or-flight response, 13, 28, 118,
    122, 129
fluoxetine (Prozac), 31, 61, 72
fluvoxamine (Luvox), 72
Freud, Anna, 29
Freud, Sigmund, 29–30, 33–34

generalized anxiety disorder (GAD),
    36, 41, 42, 92, 213
  diagnostic criteria for, 203–204
  school anxiety and, 140, 151–153
genetics, anxiety and, 15, 27, 51–52,
    86–87, 148–149
girls, 2, 11, 27, 43–44
glossary, 213–214
goals, 95–100, 112, 196–202
  charts for, 98, 99, 101

exercise and, 144
realistic, 200–201
step-wise progression of, 135

home schooling, 134–135

imagery, 122, 128–130. *See also*
    relaxation techniques
imipramine (Tofranil), 61, 72

Journal, xiv–xv, 3–4, 7, 145, 156
  alternatives to writing in, 9, 85
  charts for recording thoughts,
      109–110
  for cognitive restructuring, 153
  goal setting and, 100–101
  illustrations for, 119, 156
  to list resources, 162
  medication recorded in, 120
  for pre-readers, 105
  recording relaxation practice, 130
  scoring anxiety level in, 84–90

Klein, Donald, 61
Klonopin (clonazepam), 67, 71, 74

Letter to Kids, xiii–xv
Lexapro (escitalopram), 72
Librium (chlordiazepoxide), 60
lorazepam (Ativan), 67, 71
Luvox (fluvoxamine), 72

medication, 31, 54–56, 59–64,
    76–77, 120. *See also* therapy;
    *individual names of drugs*
  addiction/dependence on, 68
  antidepressants, 31, 33, 61–63, 69,
      71–73
  benzodiazepines, 60–64, 67, 69,
      71–74
  delayed symptom relief from, 73
  determining need for, 65–66,
      70–74, 119–120
  episodic use of, 55–56
  immediate symptom relief from,
      66–69
  relaxation and, 117–123

medication *(continued)*
for school anxiety, 139
side effects of, 63, 67
memory, 106
mental disorders
assessing, 97
diagnosing, 34
medication and, 62
resources, 218
mind-body connectedness, 117
mirtazapine (Remeron), 72
mortality rates, 179

National Alliance for the Mentally
Ill—Children and Adolescents
Network (NAMICAN), 218

National Institute of Mental Health,
218
nefazodone (Serzone), 72, 73
negative outlook, 44
nervousness, defined, 213
nortriptyline (Pamelor), 72–73

obsessive-compulsive disorder
(OCD), 36, 39–41, 213–214
cognitive behavioral treatment for,
111
diagnostic criteria for, 206–207
example, 115–117, 148–151
Obsessive Compulsive Foundation, 218
school anxiety and, 140
Specific Anxiety Disorder Inventory, 92
Oklahoma City bombing. *See*
terrorism
overanxious disorder, 30

Pamelor (nortriptyline), 72–73
panic attacks, 12–15, 214. *See also*
panic disorder; panic disorder
with agoraphobia
criteria for, 203
examples, 131–133
imipramine (Tofranil) for, 61
response to, 48

spontaneous *vs.* situational, 17, 23
triggers for, 159–162
panic disorder, 214. *See also* panic
disorder with agoraphobia
school anxiety and, 139–143
social phobia *vs.*, 145
panic disorder with agoraphobia,
36–38
diagnostic criteria for, 210–211
Specific Anxiety Disorder Inventory, 92
parents. *See also* adults
as allies, 107
anxiety in, 27, 54, 94, 184–185
blamed for children's anxiety, 30,
51
family team strategy, 53–54, 56,
169–175
praise from, 107, 118, 201–202
reaction of, 15–16, 47–50, 84–90,
108, 169–175
teaching children about risk, 178,
183
paroxetine (Paxil), 31, 61, 72
parties, 124–125
pathological anxiety, 14, 16, 193
Paxil (paroxetine), 31, 61, 72
phobias, 24–25, 214. *See also* fear;
specific phobia
physical illness
breathlessness and, 163
caused by anxiety, 70, 143–145
fear of, 74–75
preventing, 86
play dates, 124–125, 134
positive outlook, 44
posttraumatic stress disorder
(PTSD), 36, 42, 48
diagnostic criteria for, 204–206
school anxiety and, 154–156
serotonin reuptake inhibitors for,
62
Specific Anxiety Disorder Inventory, 92
practice, defined, 213
practice charts, 112–113
preschool-aged children, 105, 199